# INTRODUCTION TO
# HOMEOPATHIC MEDICINE

# Introduction to Homeopathic Medicine

HAMISH W. BOYD, M.D.

MB, ChB, FRCP(Glas), DCH, FFHom

Keats Publishing, Inc.  New Canaan, Connecticut

**Note:** The spelling of homeopathy herein follows the British style as it appears in the original text. Where new material has been added (cover text, bibliography, introductory copy, list of companies making and selling homeopathic products, etc.), Americanized spelling has been used.

To my father, William E. Boyd, MA, MD,
a wise physician and a dedicated scientist.

# Preface

For many years I have felt that we require a textbook of homoeopathic medicine, which includes principles and Materia Medica in one volume, and which sets down the procedure for case-taking and practical application of remedies. I have attempted in this book to fill such a need.

Apart from some case-taking illustrations, I have purposely omitted descriptions of patients and clinical results, which are excellently presented in books such as Margaret Tyler's *Drug Pictures* and Margery Blackie's *The Patient not the Cure*, and in the older volumes of Kent, Clarke and Nash. This book is not an attempt to convince or convert the sceptic, but to guide the interested doctor in his efforts to understand the basic principles of homoeopathy, and to help him to put these into practice.

In spite of the tremendous advances in scientific knowledge, and their application to our understanding of the workings of the human body in health and disease, there are many who feel that the Art of Medicine has largely disappeared. Suppressing or removing symptoms does not necessarily constitute cure. Cure of a patient is restoring him to a sense of well-being, physical, emotional and mental, which allows him to contribute to the full in his own life and that of the community in which he lives.

Many doctors are concerned about the treatment of their patients with some of our present-day drugs. Other forms of treatment such as hypnosis, acupuncture, herbalism, osteopathy or psychotherapy are now being studied in a search for additional ways of helping people.

Homoeopathic medicine is attracting more and more attention from patients and doctors alike, because they see in it a safe and effective form of treatment, which studies the person as a whole, with particular emphasis on him as an individual. It is not a substitute for conventional medicine, but a system of therapeutics, which enlarges and broadens the physician's outlook, and in many situations finds a real cure not possible with our usual drugs.

A good homoeopathic doctor should be a good physician first, and then a knowledgeable homoeopath.

In many situations the patient or doctor is referred to as he or him. This has been done for simplicity, and in most cases could equally well apply to the female sex.

A selection of questions for reflection and discussion are included at the end of the book. These are largely drawn from questions used in the Faculty of Homoeopathy examinations. I hope they will stimulate further reading, and assist doctors who wish to study for this qualification. A glossary of the terms used in homoeopathy is also given at the end of the book, and may prove useful for reference.

I acknowledge with grateful thanks the help I have received from the following persons: the late Dr D. M. Gibson, who gave me permission to use parts of his booklets; Dr Margery Blackie, for all she has taught me over the years, with her vivid descriptions of patients and remedies; Dr R. A. F. Jack, for his help with Accident and Injury Remedies; and Dr R. D. Calcott, for his help with Eye Remedies. I should also like to express my appreciation of valuable comments and criticisms from many colleagues on earlier drafts of the manuscript; in particular from Dr Michael Jenkins, Dr George Burns, Dr Frank Johnson, Dr Anne Clover, Dr Muir Gray and Dr Anne Bennett. I should also like to thank Mrs J. D. MacDonald for her patience in repeatedly typing and re-typing the text as alterations and new ideas were added; Mrs Brenda Marshall for the care with which she copy-edited the final draft of the manuscript; and John Churchill, my publisher, for guidance and encouragement in preparing this book. We are also indebted to the Scottish Homoeopathic Research and Educational Trust for financial assistance towards publishing.

H.W.B.

# Contents

**MATERIA  MEDICA**

SECTION I

# PRINCIPLES AND PRACTICE
# OF HOMOEOPATHY

# Chapter 1

# *What is Homoeopathy?*

Homoeopathy is a system of therapeutics for treating people and animals on the basis of the simile principle. The word 'homoeopathy' is derived from the Greek words *homoios* meaning like or similar, and *pathos* meaning suffering.

> *'Similia similibus curentur.'*
> 'Let likes be treated by likes.'

But what does this really mean?

In conventional medicine we are taught to think in terms of disease or pathological states, changes from the normal physiological state as a result of outside factors such as infection, trauma or stress, and also conditions arising from allergy or even auto-immunity. In order to treat such disease states we try to make a diagnosis based on symptoms and physical signs. This may enable us to find a cause for which there is a specific treatment or, failing this, to treat the patient's complaints by symptomatic measures.

Although there is now an increasing emphasis on the importance of treating the patient as a whole, medicine in actual fact becomes increasingly fragmented and specialised, and there are few treatments which do cure the patient as a whole.

If we look more closely at our patient we find that, although symptoms of disease fall into a variety of categories which are more or less well-defined, enabling the physician to label the disease or make a diagnosis, there are other symptoms also present. These vary from case to case, and are unique to that person. Thus, no one case, even of a well-defined disease like pneumonia, exactly resembles another, any more than two individuals are ever absolutely identical. In other words, the symptoms and signs are modified by the reaction of the patient himself.

When a plant tincture, toxic substance or 'drug' is administered in repeated doses to a group of healthy persons, certain symptoms and signs of toxicity are produced. Some of these are common to many 'drugs', and a few are characteristic of that particular 'drug'. By careful recording it is possible to build up a symptom-complex which is unique to each 'drug'. This is known as 'proving'.

The initial and all-important generalisation of Hahnemann was based on the fact that when the symptom-complex presented by the patient is compared with the symptom-complexes produced by 'drugs', in many cases there will be found a resemblance, often extraordinarily close, between the patient's symptom picture and the picture of the effects of *some* 'drug' on healthy persons.

The *basis* of homoeopathy is that the most successful remedy for any given occasion will be that one whose symptomatology presents the clearest and closest resemblance to the symptom-complex of the sick person in question.

i.e. Let likes be treated by likes.

To give a simple illustration: the effects of peeling an onion are very similar to the symptoms of acute coryza. The remedy prepared from Allium Cepa (the red onion) is used to treat the type of cold in which the symptoms resemble those we get from peeling onions.

The symptoms and signs of acute arsenic poisoning are very similar to the symptoms seen in certain cases of gastroenteritis. Arsenicum is used to treat such cases, not because the patient has taken arsenic, but because the symptoms and signs in the patient are similar to those found in arsenic overdosage.

Whenever we treat a sick person by using a method or a drug which can *cause* a similar picture in other persons, we apply the homoeopathic principle, even if we do it unconsciously.

In conventional medicine we use X-rays and radium, which cause cancer, to treat it also. We use amphetamine in the hyperactive child, although it is normally a stimulant.

Some of the treatments for immunological and allergic reactions are dependent on the use of tissue products or sera derived from infected or sensitised individuals, to produce a response in the patient to that very infection or sensitising agent. Could it be that the similar (or homoeopathy) is used more widely than we realise?

Table 1.1 sets down the two requirements for selecting a similar remedy. On the one hand there is the patient with his clinical history, his personal characteristics and his temperament, and on the other hand there is the 'drug picture' or Materia Medica. This is made up from our knowledge of toxicology, the symptoms and signs obtained from 'proving' remedies on healthy people, and symptoms added to the Materia Medica as a result of clinical observation and experience. So the first and fundamental principle of homoeopathy is the selection and use of the similar remedy.

TABLE 1.1     SELECTION OF THE SIMILAR REMEDY

| a) *The symptom picture* | b) *The 'drug' picture* |
|---|---|
| Physical characteristics | Toxicology |
| Local and general symptoms | Provings |
| Temperament of the patient | Experience |

The other, and indeed much more controversial issue, is the use of remedies in what are apparently extremely small quantities. It should be pointed out that this *use* of what are called *potentised remedies* is an extension of the method evolved by Hahnemann from experiment, and *is not in itself homoeopathy*. The use of the term 'homoeopathic' dose by doctors and scientists, usually in a derogatory or jocular fashion to denote an impossibly small quantity of some drug, is a totally inaccurate use of the term 'homoeopathic', which refers to the simile principle and not to the size of the dose. The method of preparation of remedies is described in Chapter 6, where it will be seen that a potentised remedy is not simply a very dilute solution but a scientifically and accurately prepared remedy.

Homoeopathic practice, however, is not only a question of administering remedies according to the simile principle. In order to do this successfully the homoeopathic physician must develop a different approach to his patient, one which not only seeks to make a diagnosis but also studies the patient as a whole individual, with his or her particular reaction to the causative factors of the illness.

In the course of medical teaching there is often a failure to emphasise that symptoms result not only from causal factors such as trauma, infection, malnutrition and emotional stress, but also from the reaction of the patient's own cells and tissue fluids. The way in which a person reacts to outside factors will vary from case to case, depending on that individual's physical and mental make-up. This explains the puzzling observation that two patients with the same diagnostic label may react in a totally different way, indeed the one may recover and the other die.

The way in which a homoeopathic remedy acts is still unknown, but we should always remember that the recovery of the patient depends just as much on the body's defence mechanism as it does on the drugs we give him, in most cases more so. We know more now about immunity, antibodies, hormonal and autonomic responses, but we still do not know what makes a person feel well. Cure does not consist merely of removal of symptoms, but in a full restoration of the person's physical, mental and spiritual well-being.

Hahnemann talked of the 'vital force' in human life, and it is this we must stimulate.

The persistence of homoeopathy over the last 150 years, in spite of ridicule and opposition, is proof of its effectiveness in helping sick people, even without, as yet, a scientific explanation for its action. The concept that the stimulus of the remedy triggers off a response, or bridges a gap in a metabolic or nerve reaction, seems a reasonable explanation in the light of clinical observation.

# Chapter 2

# *The Origins of Homoeopathy*

Homoeopathy was developed and given a scientific basis by Dr Samuel Hahnemann. He was born in Meissen in 1755 and his father was a painter in porcelain. Times were bad but he was determined to be a doctor. He set off for Leipzig at the age of twenty with little money in his pocket, but with the ability to speak eight languages. By means of teaching and translating scientific articles he was able to support himself until he qualified. He then quickly rose to fame, and became known as one of the most distinguished physicians in Germany. However, he saw many faults in medicine as it was then practised and did not fear to make his views known. He saw the insane treated with bodily chastisement and wrote: 'The physician in charge of such unhappy people must have at his command an attitude which inspires respect but also creates confidence.'

The overcrowding, dirt and lack of fresh air in the towns were, he thought, the cause of the epidemics. His plans for isolation hospitals, wider streets and houses with gardens were ahead of his time, and in line with modern teaching. As he practised, he became more and more dissatisfied with the methods of his day, such as bleedings, purgings and blunderbuss prescriptions. He felt that these methods did more harm than good. He decided to give himself to translating scientific literature, even though it meant giving up luxury and living in poverty.

He was asked to translate Cullen's *Materia Medica* into German. Having practised in a swampy district, the prevalent 'fever' was known by Hahnemann to respond to cinchona bark (quinine). Cullen defended the old idea that the action of cinchona on the fever was due to its tonic effect on the stomach. Not so, wrote Hahnemann to Cullen. From practical experience he knew that the strongest mixture of astringents and bitters had no effect on the fever, but such things as strong coffee, pepper, ignatia bean and arsenic did have some effect. Cullen did not reply, but Hahnemann went on wondering how it did act and decided to take some cinchona bark himself. He was amazed to find that he developed all the symptoms of the 'fever', but without pyrexia. These symptoms disappeared when he stopped taking it. After an interval he tried it again on himself, and on some of his family. All produced the same symptoms, varying only in degree. Here was a strange phenomenon; a remedy that was effective for disease, which when given to a healthy person induced the symptoms of that disease. Could there be some natural method of cure here upon which he had stumbled? He went back to the ancient literature and found that Hippocrates and, after him, Paracelsus, mentioned that substances that produced symptoms could also cure them. Hahnemann now started on his life's work.

## RESEARCH

We homoeopaths are often criticised for not having behind us a lot of research, but Hahnemann now began his research to record the effect of a large number of substances on the human body. He gathered a band of willing helpers to whom he gave remedies, and interrogated them daily on any special sensations experienced. He called these 'provings' of the remedy. One remedy was given to a number of 'provers' (healthy persons of both sexes) in repeated daily doses of small quantity and, in later trials, of actual potencies – solutions subjected to serial dilution with shaking (or 'succussion') between each stage. The provers were asked to note in a diary any symptoms and signs they experienced, particularly those which differed from their normal sensations, and symptoms which were strange or unusual. Their reports were discussed and expanded by further questioning, until a very full account was recorded of the symptoms and signs which that remedy could produce. In this way he built up a Materia Medica consisting of symptoms that he had experimentally produced in healthy people. This Materia Medica represented a vast collection of accurate observations. When identified in a sick person, they became the indication of the remedy which, given homoeopathically, would and did cure. With this Materia Medica he started medical practice once more, giving the remedy that had produced the symptoms similar to those of the disease. In its provings Belladonna had all the signs and symptoms of scarlet fever, so he gave it in an epidemic, with spectacular results. He also found that he had a prophylactic as well as a cure; the one child in a large family who escaped scarlet fever had been taking Belladonna beforehand for some other reason.

In practice he found that after a small but material dose of the indicated remedy the symptoms were aggravated before any improvement started. However, by diluting and succussing the remedy he found the improvement started with less aggravation. He called this 'potentising', and the process is described in detail in Chapter 6.

After thinking, deducing and experimenting, he presented his views and the results of his labours to the profession:

> I believe I have discovered a system which will render the practice of medicine certain and its success brilliant. I have laboured fifteen years to test my discovery – my own experiments and the testimony furnished by the records of medicine convince me of its truth. I lay it and them before you, my colleagues, and I conjure you in the name of truth, in the interest of humanity, to investigate it candidly and without prejudice.

## REACTION TO HOMOEOPATHY

How did they react? With bitter aspersions upon his personal character, contempt and scorn on the system he had unfolded, without a single suggestion to investigate or put it to the test. But having satisfied himself of the value of his discovery he battled on for the rest of his life against opposition from the medical profession, and with an ever-growing number of grateful patients.

In 1812, when the survivors of Napoleon's retreat from Moscow drifted back across Europe, they brought the scourge of typhus fever. 'Hahnemann's fame was widespread and he achieved cures bordering on the incredible.' (Hartmann, 1814.) He healed 180 cases with only one fatality.

The cholera epidemic invaded Europe eighteen years later, and again his hypothesis was shown to work. One of Hahnemann's pupils had only six deaths among 154 cholera patients. In the same town, of 1500 patients treated by the orthodox methods, 55 per cent died.

Homoeopathy spread to Britain, and there was an attempt by the medical profession to have its practice forbidden by law. A cholera epidemic came to the rescue in 1854. When it was over, the results of treatment in the various hospitals were put before Parliament. Fortunately, a homoeopathic patient was there and asked why those of the homoeopathic hospital had not been included, and demanded that they be procured. They came accompanied by a letter from the Government Inspector. The death rate was 16.4 per cent compared with 51.8 per cent at other hospitals. (These figures are confirmed in the British

Museum's records.) He said that they were all true cases of cholera, and he had seen cases recover who would have died in other hospitals. He ended by saying: 'If it should please the Lord to visit me with cholera I would wish to fall into the hands of a homoeopathic physician'.

Hahnemann, having thought through his new methods, published a book called *The Organon*, in which he recorded his thoughts. He had come to the conclusion that there was in man a balancing mechanism which kept him in perfect health, in spite of all the stresses of life (psychological, physical and atmospheric), provided that the stresses were not too great or prolonged, and that the balancing mechanism itself, which he called the 'vital force', was not impaired. But if the stress was too great, or the vital force impaired, unusual signs, sensations and symptoms followed. These were the language of the sick body. The sick body could be restored rapidly to its original state of health by a potentised remedy that had been found by experience to produce a similar condition in a healthy body.

Today a great deal is talked about stress as the cause of ill health, but there is no clear method for treating it. The results of psychological stress are often dealt with by psychiatrists and social workers. To Hahnemann the 'mental symptoms', i.e. those concerned with temperament, emotion, feelings and will, were the most important in guiding him to the correct remedy.

Hippocrates had noticed that 'disease is eliminated through remedies able to produce similar symptoms', but it was left to Hahnemann, nearly 2000 years later, to rediscover this fact for himself, and by a new method of research on the healthy human being, to develop a new pharmacy and a new method of therapeutics. All over the world this method is still practised by qualified doctors.

The idea that the body itself might be aided and abetted in its endeavours to cure the disorder and disharmony responsible for disease may have seemed ridiculous and scarcely worthy of attention to the men of Hahnemann's generation. It is by no means so absurd today, with our knowledge of immunology, allergy, molecular biology and even submolecular physics. Time and the advance of science are proving to be on Hahnemann's side.

In other respects too Hahnemann's thinking was ahead of his time. He postulated the theory that disease was in most cases not merely local but systemic, that local symptoms were but outward and visible signs of inward metabolic dysfunction, and that many so-called acute illnesses were but a flare-up or exacerbation of a deep-seated chronic disorder.

In consequence he argued that in treating an illness it is the whole person who should be considered, and not just the local manifestations of the trouble.

## REFERENCES

*Samuel Hahnemann: His Life and Work*      Richard Haehl.
*Homoeopathy*      G. Ruthven Mitchell.

# Chapter 3

# *What Does Homoeopathy Offer?*

Many people think of homoeopathic treatment as a last resort for difficult or resistant chronic illnesses, for which many other forms of treatment have already been tried. While some dramatic cures can be achieved on occasion with homoeopathy, many cases of advanced chronic illness can also be modified or helped to a limited extent. I am thinking here of conditions such as severe rheumatoid arthritis or osteoarthritis, motor neurone disease, multiple sclerosis, muscular dystrophy, leukaemias, and certain forms of cancer and severe mental illness. It is still well worth treating these conditions with homoeopathic remedies, selected on an individual basis, and taking into account the patient's total symptom picture and mental and physical characteristics as described later, rather than the purely presenting local symptoms. In this way the disease can be modified, occasionally stopped, and above all the patient's well-being and quality of life can be improved. In cases of cancer, the amount of sedation and analgesia can often be greatly reduced and the patient kept alert and comfortable, even if the ultimate result is the same. Most homoeopathic doctors would recommend surgical treatment of an early operable cancer, where this offers a good prospect of cure.

## CONDITIONS WHERE CONVENTIONAL TREATMENT IS ESSENTIAL

**Surgery**
Surgery is essential for removal of mechanical lesions, obstruction, stones, acute appendix, certain inflammatory bowel conditions, tumours and of course repair of congenital defects or orthopaedic problems. In some cases of peptic ulcer, colitis, cholecystitis and renal calculi a homoeopathic remedy will effect a cure without the need for surgery. We also believe that remedies like Arnica, Causticum, Staphisagria and Carbo Veg. can help the patient to recover more quickly and smoothly after surgery.

**Deficiencies**

Where a patient requires replacement therapy with iron, vitamin $B_{12}$, thyroxine, insulin or hormones, the appropriate treatment with a conventional drug is given in normal dosage.

In gross cardiac and renal failure, and biochemical imbalance, orthodox treatment will usually be necessary, but can be successfully supplemented by homoeopathic remedies.

**Severe infections**

In active pulmonary tuberculosis, venereal diseases, meningitis and severe septicaemia most homoeopathic doctors would advocate the use of antibiotics along with homoeopathic remedies.

## WHERE THEN DOES HOMOEOPATHY HAVE ITS GREATEST FIELD OF ACTION?

Undoubtedly in the field of *primary care.*

In hospital practice as a young doctor or student we often get the impression that we can cure many illnesses, and do some dramatic things. It is only when we get out into the field of general practice that we realise many conditions are still very difficult to treat: allergies, skin conditions, rheumatism and arthritis, asthma, migraine, and of course the wide range of psychosomatic illnesses, and people who are merely not well.

There is increasing concern on the part of both lay and medical men and women at the amount of illness caused by overprescribing, by side effects and by reactions occurring in sensitive individuals. In general practice only a small percentage of patients suffer from clear cut diagnostic disease, or conditions which can be treated successfully with all the latest drugs. Doctors who come to study homoeopathy are very often individualists, concerned about the quantity of sedatives, tranquillisers, antispasmodics and antibiotics they are prescribing, and seeking safer and more effective ways of helping their patients. Homoeopathy is not a panacea, but it is of immense value in treating many common ailments.

**First aid and injury**

There are a number of useful remedies for emergency use in these situations, which can be given either by a doctor or equally well by a lay person in the home or at work. These are described more fully in

Section II (Chapter 9), the common ones being Aconite, Arnica, Rhus Tox., Calendula, Hypericum and Ledum.

**Acute infections and respiratory disease**

Although antibiotics have revolutionised acute bacterial infections, the problem of acquired resistance by organisms is well known, and a constant stream of new antibiotics flood the market from the pharmaceutical industry. Side effects can occur with most of these drugs, and others cause allergic reactions in sensitive individuals. The bowel flora is disturbed and fungal infections occur. Antibiotics should be selected with care and only used if absolutely essential.

Homoeopathic remedies will clear up many sore throats, fevers, coughs and septic lesions without the use of an antibiotic, by helping to stimulate the body's natural defence mechanisms to overcome the infection. They are particularly useful in children with recurring chest infections or tonsillitis, where an antibiotic clears up the acute phase and then relapse occurs within a week or two. We as doctors and also as parents are often concerned at the amount of antibiotics sometimes given to these children. They may develop chronic catarrh, secretory otitis media, deafness or discharging ears; their adenoids, tonsils and glands become enlarged and sometimes operation becomes necessary. Homoeopathic remedies can often reduce catarrh, greatly improve the child's health, and avoid these complications. As stated earlier we should seek to find a remedy for that individual child based on his total symptom picture and personality, and not just a local remedy. Chapter 20 on children's remedies describes a number of the useful ones for different types of children, such as Calc. Carb., Pulsatilla, Sulphur and Silica.

We should also never forget in these children the problem of house dust or animal allergy, which is often the cause of their wheeze or catarrh rather than an infection. Again these can be helped by homoeopathic vaccines of the allergens, together with appropriate preventive measures against house dust mite.

*Influenza*

This and certain associated virus diseases, which are virtually unaffected by known orthodox drugs, have responded over the years to the indicated remedy such as Gelsemium, Eupatorium, Rhus Tox., Baptisia and Pyrogen (Chapter 12).

*Pneumonia*

This was successfully treated by homoeopathy long before the advent of antibiotics. Homoeopathic remedies are still effective, although sometimes an antibiotic is used in addition, in a feeble patient or for a severe infection.

*Asthma*

This requires careful study to find the causative factors. Some patients may require Intal or Ventolin, or in extreme cases steroids, but there are several valuable acute homoeopathic remedies for asthmatic attacks. Even more important, the patient should be treated between attacks by a constitutional remedy, which will improve his health and reduce the incidence and severity of the attacks, and in many cases completely abolish them.

**Gastrointestinal illness**

In Chapter 13 you will find a number of remedies which will cure or alleviate acute diarrhoea and vomiting, dyspepsia, peptic ulcer, colitis (particularly irritable bowel syndrome and even some cases of ulcerative colitis), and piles. There are few specifics in homoeopathy, and each case must be individualised to find the best remedy in that situation. The wrong remedy will not cure.

**Rheumatism and arthritis**

This group of diseases is one of the main causes of disability and loss of working hours. Many of these patients have no obvious pathological change, and merely complain of pain and stiffness, sometimes related to the weather. Homoeopathic remedies will cure these. Where there is advanced bony change and joint damage, the best one can hope for is some alleviation and improved mobility. Here again homoeopathy can do a great deal. It can reduce the amount of analgesics and antirheumatic drugs, and often help where the patient cannot tolerate these drugs due to side effects and allergic reactions. Good physiotherapy, occupational therapy and occasionally surgery are also important (Chapter 17).

**Headaches**

It is essential to exclude severe pathological lesions, like neoplasm or arterial disease, which may require neurosurgery, but the vast majority of headaches are due either to migraine or to psychological stresses and tension. In homoeopathy we have a number of acute headache remedies, selected on the basis of their modalities (factors which modify the pain like heat, cold, pressure, movement, etc.). These are described in Chapter 10.

Even more important, as in asthma, we should try to treat the patient between attacks with a carefully selected general remedy which suits that individual. In this way we can reduce the incidence and severity of attacks, and in many cases clear them up altogether.

## Skin conditions

It is important to distinguish between external causes of skin disease such as scabies or pediculosis, where a local application will cure the condition, and eczema, dermatitis and psoriasis. These are often skin manifestations of a general underlying problem, due either to heredity, allergies or emotional stress. Here the homoeopath will try to treat the patient rather than the skin, and will use a minimum of local ointments, especially steroids. The concept of suppression of skin disease resulting in more deep-seated internal illness is discussed elsewhere (pages 31 and 55); many doctors have observed an eczema or dermatitis apparently clearing up with local applications, but in fact being suppressed, and being followed by asthma or gastric symptoms.

Remedies for shingles are also discussed in the section on skin. Rhus Tox. and Ranunculus Bulb. will often act very quickly, relieving the burning pain and encouraging rapid healing (Chapter 16).

## Genito-urinary disease

Although a large or impacted calculus may require surgery, the remedy Berberis will often relieve the pain of renal colic and encourage passage of a stone. Acute cystitis may on occasions require an antibiotic, especially in younger patients where there is proven bacterial infection, but remedies like Cantharis, Causticum and Terebinth are often all that is required. The problem of recurring attacks of cystitis or chronic infection is a difficult one in practice, and here the homoeopathic remedy for the patient is often of value, or a bowel nosode like Sycotic Co. Prescribing in this way will reduce the need for repeated antibiotics and, in some patients, stop the relapses entirely.

There are a number of remedies for the treatment of leucorrhoea, dysmenorrhoea and the symptoms of the menopause, but these should be selected for the individual patient based on her general and mental symptoms, and not merely on the local pain or discharge. Where there is a large fibroid or ovarian cyst, or an obvious prolapse, surgery may be indicated (Chapter 15).

**Cardiovascular disease**

Where a patient has cardiac irregularities or gross heart failure, drugs like Digoxin or diuretics may be necessary, and in acute myocardial infarction intensive care may be required; but there are many valuable remedies in homoeopathy for angina and heart failure, such as Crataegus, Cactus, Carbo Veg. and Lachesis. Patients with hypertension should always be given their constitutional remedies and tinctures like Crataegus before resorting to diuretics, beta-blocking drugs or other antihypertensive agents, particularly if they are elderly. Many doctors are still not convinced that merely lowering the readings of a sphygmomanometer makes the patient feel better, or improves long term prognosis.

In cases of cerebrovascular accident, remedies like Arnica, Opium and Gelsemium can sometimes bring about remarkable improvement (Chapter 14).

**Psychosomatic illness and anxiety states**

In general practice there are a large number of patients who present with illness resulting from stress, emotional upsets or environmental situations, and these may cause nervous symptoms or even physical signs. While discussion of the patient's problems and an attempt to solve the causal factors undoubtedly helps, a suitable homoeopathic constitutional remedy can also be of value. It will be seen that the homoeopathic method of case-taking, with its detail and emphasis on temperamental symptoms, may well play a valuable psychological part in aiding recovery, although this should be a part of all medical history-taking if time allows. While there is an awareness of the need for preventive medicine, and of a positive attitude to health as opposed to disease, there is often no suitable remedy which can be prescribed before pathological changes have started. We firmly believe that homoeopathic remedies can deal with illness in its early stages, and perhaps prevent the development of more serious disease.

Only a brief summary has been given in this survey of possible fields of use for homoeopathy. There is almost no situation in which a homoeopathic remedy is not of some value, except perhaps in some instances where the patient is receiving intensive medication with several potent conventional drugs.

The homoeopathic doctor seldom, if ever, says to a patient, 'There is nothing more I can do for you'. Always he is searching for a better remedy and a fuller understanding of his patient, and of that person's need. Every patient is an individual problem, with his own unique personality and reaction, and not just 'a case of bronchitis or colitis'. It is perfectly possible to combine homoeopathy with conventional medicine in many situations, but with increasing experience the doctor will find himself using less of the palliative drugs, and more homoeopathy, with the satisfaction of curing his patients in the true sense.

It should be stated firmly that homoeopathy does not consist of using conventional drugs in inadequate dosage. Where a conventional drug, analgesic, sedative, antibiotic or cardiac drug is used by a homoeopathic doctor, it is used in the correct orthodox dose. Only homoeopathic potencies are given in their specially prepared dilutions.

In Section II you will find remedies grouped under the body systems, with descriptions of the leading symptoms for each remedy on which to prescribe. Some doctors will find these a useful starting point for prescribing, until they have grasped the concept of remedies for 'people' rather than 'diseases'.

# Chapter 4

# *The Materia Medica*

Mention was made in Chapter 2 of the 'proving' of remedies, the method whereby symptoms and signs of minor or major toxicity, from administering repeated small doses of a substance to healthy volunteers, were collected and assessed.

This 'proving' has continued over the years, using a wide variety of substances. Tinctures of plants, salts, metals, venoms of snakes and spiders, and even certain synthetic drugs have all been 'proved', and their symptoms and signs recorded and assessed. In addition, the known toxicology of each substance has been added. A third group of symptoms and signs – those which have been helped or cured by the particular remedy in a reasonable number of patients – have been included.

These three groups make up the detailed Materia Medica used by the homoeopathic physician. They form the symptom-complex characteristic of the remedy (see Table 1.1, page 4).

1 Poisoning and toxicology
2 Provings
3 Experiential symptoms

In addition to these factual records, observations have enabled physicians to associate certain characteristics of appearance and temperament with the effectiveness of particular remedies. This makes it possible to select a suitable remedy for the patient by taking into account his whole physical and mental make-up, in addition to the detailed analysis of his symptoms.

It is difficult for a conventionally trained physician to think of a remedy or drug having a symptom picture. We think of a drug having a certain chemical composition, causing particular effects on body physiology or pathology, and being used for a specific purpose or disease. However, every drug does produce side effects or toxic reactions, and it is these which the homoeopathic doctor takes note of and uses as a part of his Materia Medica. Most of the remedies used in homoeopathy are derived from *naturally* occurring substances – whole plants, minerals and salts – and not from single extracts or refined synthetic products. This does not mean that a 'pure' synthetic drug cannot be used homoeopathically, but a fresh 'proving' would have to be carried out to find the 'drug picture' of that substance. It is for this reason that we retain the Latin name for a remedy, such as Natrum Muriaticum, instead of calling it Sodium Chloride, which would infer a purified product. The source of Natrum Mur. is described in the pharmacopoeia, and the remedy of that name is known throughout the world in any language.

## THE REMEDY PICTURE

Each remedy in the Materia Medica contains a description of the symptoms and signs associated with it, set out under the systems of the body. These vary from apparently minor symptoms to gross toxic effects, the amount of detail depending on the text. One of the characteristic features of a homoeopathic Materia Medica is the inclusion of modalities of symptoms. These are things which qualify a symptom, for example the type of pain and what things make it better or worse: movement, rest, heat, cold, damp, time of day. In addition to local symptoms, we find general symptoms affecting the person as a whole, and mental symptoms related to the temperament, emotions and feelings. It is necessary in studying a remedy to memorise as much as possible of the characteristics of that particular remedy, which organs it affects, and also to note if there is one kind of symptom running through the various systems. For example, in Bryonia we find marked dryness and aggravation from movement appearing in many local areas, or cramping pains in Cuprum, or stitching pains in Kali Carb.

Examples of prominent features in certain remedies are:

Aconitum: Acuteness of onset, extreme restlessness, marked terror, intense thirst.

Belladonna: Bright red face, bounding pulse, burning hot skin, staring eyes with widely dilated pupils, a bellicose type of delirium.

Sulphur: Widespread burnings, disturbances of circulation, marked intolerance of heat.

A similar set of symptoms can be found in patients, and details of this are explained in the next chapter on case-taking. It is the matching of these two sets of symptoms in patient and remedy which is the essence of homoeopathic prescribing; in other words, the selection of the similar remedy.

Because of the great number of remedies and symptoms, doctors using homoeopathy have compiled dictionaries or 'repertories'. These show what symptoms are present in different remedies, and indicate their importance. The best known repertories are those of Kent, Boenninghausen, Boericke and Clarke, and more recently the *Synthetic Repertory* of Barthel and Klunker. Card repertories are now in use by Kishore and Brousallian and Flury, and the information from many of these is being put on to computer tape and disc, with a view to simplifying remedy selection.

In using a repertory it is necessary to take a careful case history, to select the symptoms which are most prominent, along with their modalities, and then to look these up under the system affected, e.g. general, mind, extremities, stomach, cough, bladder, etc. Here you will find symptoms described in the patient's words and a number of remedies in different type. The remedies in heaviest type are the most important to consider. By studying a number of symptoms, certain remedies will be seen to come through strongly, and these should be studied further in the Materia Medica to obtain the best selected remedy.

Whilst it is of obvious interest to know the origin of the remedy, it is also helpful from the point of view of treatment, for remedies fall into groups – botanical, chemical, biological – and members of a group are often complementary in action. They will follow each other well, and indeed enhance the effect.

This does not mean that they are interchangeable, for it is usually just one remedy that is eminently suited to the needs of the patient. But one member of the group may be able to aid and abet another, and it sometimes requires more than one remedy in series to bring about the desired cure.

Next the pharmacology of the remedy and its sources is worthy of study. It reveals affinities with particular tissues, organs or systems that render the symptoms associated with the remedy more understandable. The knowledge of these tissue or organ affinities may also be of value in prescribing. Examples are the known affinity of:

Iodum with the thyroid gland,
Chelidonium with the liver and gallbladder,
Belladonna with the central nervous system,

Cantharis with the genito-urinary system,
Rhus Toxicodendron with the locomotor system,
Ruta Graveolens with the periosteum,
Arnica with injured tissues,
Hypericum with nervous tissue,
Sepia with the female pelvic organs.

Awareness of these tissue affinities may suggest the possible use of one or more remedies, which can then be studied for suitability with other features of the individual case.

Homoeopathy studies and deals with the individual as a whole. The individual remedy must be approached, understood and known in the same way. The drug picture must be seen as a whole with its own individual features, so distinctive as to be recognised promptly when its counterpart is met in a sick person. This is an art which can only be acquired by continual study, coupled with constant observation.

## REFERENCES

*Materia Medica Pura*   Samuel Hahnemann.
*Dictionary of Practical Materia Medica*   J. H. Clarke.
*Materia Medica with Repertory*   W. Boericke.
*Lectures on Homoeopathic Materia Medica*   J. T. Kent.
*Keynotes of Leading Remedies*   M. C. Allen.
*Homoeopathic Drug Pictures*   M. L. Tyler.
*Condensed Materia Medica*   C. Hering.

## REPERTORIES

*Repertory of Homoeopathic Materia Medica*   J. T. Kent.
*Boenninghausen's Characteristics and Repertory*   Translated by C. M. Boger.
*Clinical Repertory*   J. H. Clarke.
*Practical Repertory*   R. Flury.
*Synthetic Repertory*   H. Barthel and W. Klunker.

# Chapter 5

# *Case-Taking and Diagnosis*

In many ways case-taking for the homoeopathic physician is more difficult than for his orthodox colleagues. He must not only make a diagnosis in the usual way, where this is possible, but he must also be thinking at the same time of a suitable homoeopathic remedy, based on the patient's own characteristic reaction and symptom picture.

Accurate and painstaking history-taking is at the very heart of the homoeopathic approach. Only by this can the all-important details of the particular illness and the individual characteristics of the particular patient be arrived at, matters essential for the selection of the Similar Remedy.

In the first place, every effort should be made to discover as far as possible what is going on, and what is going wrong, in the body of the sick person: what organs are diseased, what functions are deranged, what tissues are damaged or disordered.

These are pertinent questions, and the answers to them, when available, may reveal a need for surgical, dietetic, supportive or sub-stitutionary treatment. A diagnosis must be made, wherever possible. Nevertheless, the risk of being over-engrossed in the 'part' to the neglect of the 'whole' must always be borne in mind.

Knowledge of underlying pathology, in addition possibly to pointing to the need for surgical or other ancillary measures, may be of assistance to the homoeopath because of his knowledge of 'tissue affinities' (Chapter 4). The relation of certain remedies to specific organs or tissues may be of significance for therapy, when such organs or tissue are known to be involved in the disease process.

A careful *physical examination* must always be carried out after history-taking. The full facilities of modern diagnostic techniques should be utilised, when these are relevant and in the genuine interests of the patient.

## ACUTE CASE-TAKING

When presented with an acute illness the doctor should try to select a few leading symptoms and signs presented by the patient, study the modalities of these and take into account the appearance and immediate mental symptoms of the patient, in particular any change from the patient's usual temperament. This will become clearer when you study the Materia Medica in relation to acute illnesses. Such things as restlessness, fear, irritability in a normally placid individual, desire for company or wish to be left alone, thirst or its absence in a fever, as well as the modalities of the cough or pain, will enable selection of a remedy to be made rapidly with the minimum of questioning (See Table 5.1, page 33.)

In young children, the observation of the mother or nurse will be of particular value in this respect.

## CHRONIC CASE-TAKING

### The complaint and present history
Attention must first be paid to the particular symptoms of which the patient complains, both in relation to the present illness and also any other troubles. The latter may be considered of minor importance by the patient but may well be of signal significance in remedy selection.

### Onset and course of the illness
For example, a sudden onset and rapid development may point to Aconitum or Belladonna. Insidious onset and gradual progress suggest Bryonia, Gelsemium or Pulsatilla.

Enquiry must include any possible *cause* of illness, either recent or remote. The aetiological factor can be of considerable importance in pointing to a definite remedy.

A history of illness coming on quickly after exposure to severe dry cold would suggest Aconitum, Hepar Sulph. or Causticum; illness ensuing after getting chilled when hot, or after a soaking with rain, might require Dulcamara; effects of loss of sleep might point to Cocculus; a history of head injury, perhaps remote, would suggest Natrum Sulphuricum or Arnica; and so on. Aconitum may also be indicated where the history of onset dates from a bad fright or shock.

Again, the character of the pain or other symptoms must be enquired into, the sort of pain, the site, the spread, the severity and, above all, the modalities.

## Modalities

A modality is something which qualifies a symptom and often enables a choice to be made between two quite strongly indicated remedies. These may be of various kinds:

*Thermal modalities* relate to reactions to heat and cold. Heat may aggravate or give relief, cold likewise, and these effects are highly characteristic of individual remedies.

*Meteorological modalities* are of great importance, the effects of weather changes, wet, wind, thunder, sea air and the like.

*Physical modalities* such as the effects of rest, posture, active movement, passive movement, exertion, jolt or jar.

*Time modalities* refer to aggravation or relief of symptoms at a particular hour of the day or season of the year.

A further aspect sometimes comes into consideration, namely laterality. It so happens that many remedies show a relation to symptoms which are predominantly either right-sided or left-sided, or spread in a characteristic manner. For instance:

Symptoms starting on the right side and spreading to the left point to Lycopodium; those starting on the left and extending to the right indicate Lachesis; symptoms which shuttle from side to side point to Lac. Caninum; pain shooting centrally up a limb points to Hypericum; pain shooting down the limb indicates Kalmia; pain spreading in all directions points to Dioscorea.

## Past history

A history of such illnesses as asthma, eczema, hay fever, rheumatic fever, pleurisy, kidney disease, tuberculosis or venereal disease, or of previous operations is of course relevant. To the homoeopathic physician a history of injury might call for Arnica, severe reaction to smallpox vaccination might indicate the need for Thuja, or a history of never having been well since measles would suggest the use of the nosode Morbillinum.

## Family history

Knowledge of the health of parents and siblings can be helpful, not only on account of inherited illnesses, but because a history of cancer or tuberculosis might well indicate the need for Carcinosin or Tuberculinum in the patient.

Having obtained details of the patient's complaint and present history, the past and family history, we must then obtain details which will tell us more about the patient himself, his reactions and temperament. These can be classified under certain main headings.

**Physical characteristics**
Both provings and clinical observations have shown a close relationship between remedies and outstanding physical features – complexion, appearance, manner, colour, peculiarities of hair, skin, discharge, movements, posture, speech and odour.

Features which stand out are at once connected by the observer who knows his Materia Medica with a remedy which has the same features prominent in its drug picture. For example:

The tense, well-groomed, fastidious Arsenicum patient, unable to relax or stay put even at night.

The pale, podgy, phlegmatic chilly Calcarea patient.

The tall, delicate-looking, red-haired Phosphorus patient, fidgety, and nervously anxious to assist and give accurate answers when questioned.

The stoop-shouldered, rather unkempt, red-faced, talkative, self-opinionated, warm-blooded Sulphur patient.

It should be pointed out, however, that although these characteristic features may help in selecting a remedy, not every tense well-groomed person is Arsenicum, nor every red-haired patient a Phosphorus. These are merely additional guides to remedy selection.

**General symptoms**
These refer to the patient as a whole, and are features the patient exhibits even while in perfect health. How does he react to heat or cold, or to extremes of these? People vary in their thermal reactions. Nux Vomica types are excessively chilly, and hug the fire in winter. Pulsatilla persons on the other hand dislike hot weather, are ill-at-ease in a hot stuffy atmosphere, crave air and want windows widely open, get overheated in bed and push off the covers, but may before long feel chilly and pull them on again.

*Perspiration*
Does he perspire and if so where – head, feet, body? Head sweats at night, soaking the pillow, suggest Calcarea Carb. Sweaty malodorous feet could indicate Silica.

*Time*
Many patients appear to have an aggravation of their symptoms at

particular times of the day or night. If this aggravation is of a recurrent nature, for example the cough or fever is always worse in the evening, or the patient feels generally worse at that time, this may provide specific indications for the selection of the correct remedy. Some well-known times of aggravation are 1–2 a.m. (Arsenicum Album), 3–4 a.m. (Kali Carb.), 4–8 p.m. (Lycopodium), etc.

*Weather*
Does frost or damp or thunder affect him? The modalities mentioned under the local complaint may well apply also in a general sense.

*Food cravings and aversions*
These are only of value if they are strong likes or dislikes and are not influenced by advice, habit, religion or other factors.

The commonest ones of help are desire for or aversion to sweet food, sugar itself, salt, highly seasoned food, eggs, fat, milk, fish. This should be distinguished from foods which upset although desired.

Peculiarities of appetite are associated with many remedies. Natrum Muriaticum subjects are proverbially hungry, eat heartily but remain thin. Several remedies, notably Phosphorus and Sulphur, show a mid-morning empty sensation which demands a snack for relief.

Lycopodium subjects have very capricious appetites; they may feel quite hungry immediately after a meal or they may feel full after only a few mouthfuls. Desire for such things as chalk or coal suggest Calcarea Carbonica.

Food likes and dislikes vary a great deal from one person to another. Lycopodium subjects have a great preference for hot meals and very hot fluids. Phosphorus types, on the other hand, want spicy food, cold meals and even ice-cold drinks. A craving for salt strongly points to Natrum Muriaticum. Food intolerances are many, and if marked in the individual may have their counterpart under one or more remedies. When taken into account with other features in the case, all these personal peculiarities assist in arriving at and choosing a remedy that is most suitable because it is most similar on several counts.

Thirst is another aspect of some significance. Some remedies, notably Apis, Gelsemium and Pulsatilla, show absence of thirst in situations when this would not be expected, i.e. in an acute pyrexia. Natrum Muriaticum subjects are usually extremely thirsty.

A desire for frequent sips of water points to Arsenicum Album. A demand for large amounts at long intervals suggests Bryonia. Excessive thirst associated with a poor appetite points to Sulphur.

## Sleep

The pattern of sleep, position in sleep, and the type of dreams may be of value. Some patients lie awake for hours, others will sleep and then wake at 1 a.m. (Arsenicum Album), or 3–4 a.m. (Kali Carb.). The Pulsatilla child often sleeps with his hands above his head. The knee-elbow position may indicate Phosphorus or Medorrhinum. A Lachesis patient cannot bear to lie on the left side, because her heart beats strongly. Dreams may be recurring and of significance – of fire, the dead, escaping, etc. The repertory will often indicate remedies with these marked symptoms.

## Menstrual disturbances

The effect of the period on the patient's well-being as a whole is a general symptom, e.g. worse before and relieved by the flow. Variations in the appearance of the flow, types of pain and of discharge are particular symptoms.

## Mental symptoms

In selecting the correct homoeopathic remedy these symptoms rank highest in importance. The patient's personality, temperament and psychological features may be assessed to some extent by observation. Questioning may elicit such things as fears, attitude to heights or enclosed spaces, tidiness or the reverse, irritability, weepiness, a like or dislike of sympathy or of company, a tendency to worry or to become extremely upset in anticipation, sensitivity to noise and also hobbies and interests. (See also Table 5.2, page 34.)

## Mental characteristics

In these days the importance of the psychogenic aspect of disease is being realised more and more. From its inception homoeopathy has always emphasised the significance of the mental, especially the emotional features in a case-history. Many remedies are intimately related to outstanding psychological symptoms. For example:

The utter apathy and indifference of Sepia.
The jealousy of Lachesis.
The abysmal suicidal gloom of Aurum Metallicum.
The tiresomely fussy tidiness of Arsenicum.
The nervous apprehension before an ordeal of Argentum Nitricum.
The emotional instability of Ignatia.
The disdainful superiority of Platina.
The tearfulness and variability of Pulsatilla.
The intractable irritability of Chamomilla.

This whole range of temperament and mental attitudes, sensitivities and even odd sensations, as recorded under different remedies, affords pertinent pointers to their use.

With experience the doctor will learn to assess many aspects of a patient's temperament and personality merely by observing how he or she responds to questioning, the way he behaves or his mannerisms in the home or consulting room, without actually asking specific questions. He will sense whether he is outgoing and extrovert, or only giving very guarded answers. He will see if he is tearful or resentful, irritable or tidy, and in this way form a picture of the patient as a person, and hence what remedy may suit him.

**Particular symptoms**
These are symptoms related to parts, and may well have been obtained in the present history. It is important to enquire about the modalities in relation to particular symptoms, i.e. the factors which qualify a symptom, as described on page 34.

**Strange, rare and peculiar symptoms**
You may come across this term in homoeopathic literature and it is used to include inexplicable reactions. For example: asthma relieved by lying down; difficulty in swallowing liquids, while solids present no problem; symptoms with laterality or time aggravations.

**Observation**
During the taking of the patient's case history, which should be obtained with as little interruption as possible, certain observations can be made, which may greatly facilitate selection of the remedy.

*Posture*
A patient sitting tense and erect on the edge of the chair suggests Arsenicum Album. One who flops into the chair and lounges at full length, omitting perhaps to remove his hat, might point to Sulphur. One who sits there wringing her hands, probably Ignatia or Phosphorus. One with constant movements, especially of the feet, suggests the possibility of Zincum Metallicum.

*Manners*
Excited, suggests Phosphorus; apathetic, points to Sepia; obviously holding back tears, likely to be Natrum Muriaticum; haughty and disdainful, indicates Platina.

*Complexion*
Bright red face points to Belladonna; quick changes of colour would suggest Ignatia; pallor of lips, ears and fingers would indicate Calcarea Carbonica.

*Expression*
A scared panicky look points to Aconitum; a furtive glint in the eye suggests Lachesis; a bashful, bored appearance may indicate Baryta Carbonica; a deep furrow above the root of the nose typifies Lycopodium.

*Hair*
Dry, lustreless hair would suggest several remedies, among them Medorrhinum and Psorinum; sleek well-kept hair might point to Arsenicum Album; alopecia areata would suggest Phosphorus; strikingly red lips would point to Tuberculinum.

*Speech*
This is especially worthy of note; a spate of words, uttered rather disjointedly, jumping from subject to subject, points to Lachesis; pontificating conversation in the manner of the club bore strongly suggests Sulphur; readiness to reply, with perhaps some hesitation for the sake of accuracy, indicates Phosphorus.

*Clothes*
May suggest Arsenicum Album if strikingly smart and neat; the reverse, a somewhat untidy, unkempt look would point to Sulphur.

*Odour*
An offensive body odour would suggest Mercurius or Psorinum; a sour smell of discharges or stools would point to Calcarea Carbonica; a pungent cadaverous odour would suggest Baptisia; a particularly foul odour would point to Carbo Vegetabilis or Psorinum.

The remedies mentioned are just a few examples from the Materia Medica. (See also Table 5.2, pages 33—4.)


## THE CONSTITUTIONAL REMEDY

This term leads to confusion amongst those studying homoeopathy, and indeed many experienced homoeopaths use the term in rather differing ways.

We have discussed the need, wherever possible, and in particular in chronic disease, to look at the whole patient. To seek symptoms referable not just to his complaint or the particular part of the body, but also to his general reactions to weather and food, as well as seeking his mental symptoms. In this way we use the totality of symptoms to select a remedy.

Following Hahnemann, other homoeopaths, especially Kent in America and Margaret Tyler in Britain, began to introduce a further concept. This was the idea that people of a certain build, colouring or appearance, with certain distinguishable characteristics of behaviour or mannerisms, and of a certain temperament, seemed to respond to particular 'polycrest' remedies (certain frequently used remedies with a wide spectrum of clinical symptoms). So in addition to taking the actual presenting symptoms, they learned to observe and assess their patients as individuals of a particular type. We have already made comments about the Arsenic, Sulphur or Pulsatilla type. These doctors then often selected their remedy on the basis of the patient's type. This is noticeable in Borland's descriptions of children, described in Chapter 20. The concept of constitutional types has become a part of homoeopathic prescribing amongst many British physicians, although in fact it is not an original Hahnemannian idea.

Constitutional prescribing of this sort is of value in the early stages of disease, and particularly after an acute episode. It seems to build up the patient's resistance, improving his well-being and helping to prevent relapses, for example in migraine or asthma. It is also valuable in chronic disease where the main complaint is pathological, as in severe rheumatoid arthritis. Here, by seeking out the whole personality of the patient, with his fears and sensitivities, and his emotional reactions to people and environment, we can prescribe a constitutional remedy. This does not alter the basic personality of the patient but improves his health and often also his pain, stiffness and mobility as well.

Although people have a personality or belong to a type, what matters most is a change from the normal – especially in the mental sphere – increased irritability, jealousy, tearfulness or even obsessional tidiness or loss of interest. These are the symptoms to prescribe on.

Some doctors use the term 'constitutional prescribing' to describe selection of a remedy on the totality of the symptoms that tell us what the patient is like, and use the remedy intercurrently as described above. Others use the term only when they take into account the type of patient, including observation of build, colour and behaviour, as already mentioned.

I do not feel that this matters, as long as we are clear what we mean by the term. Our aim in either case is the same – to attempt to improve health and provide a sense of well-being. To effect real cure in chronic illness, these broad deep-acting remedies are essential – local prescribing will usually only palliate.

## HAHNEMANN'S THREE 'MIASMS'

Diseases can be broadly classified as acute or chronic. A true acute disease is not deep-seated and can be completely cured by a well-selected homoeopathic remedy, or will recover on its own due to the patient's natural recuperative powers. Some acute diseases seem to recur, and this may be due to the fact that they are not acute diseases as such, but acute exacerbations of an underlying chronic disease. These will not clear up with one remedy, but may need several remedies in succession, and often a constitutional remedy to follow an acute one.

Chronic diseases are a result of many factors in the patient's history, including inherited predisposition, as well as the influence of disease in parents or grandparents. We now know the importance of genetic inheritance, and the effect on a child of illness during pregnancy. Hahnemann maintained that much chronic illness was due to suppression of disease, particularly skin disease or other superficial conditions which are not truly cured by local applications and drugs, but merely suppressed, leading to more deep-seated illness. Many homoeopaths believe that suppressing eczema with steroids may cause asthma to develop, i.e. a more superficial illness is replaced by a deeper one, and that cure can occur only if diseases exteriorise. That is, the patient feels better when a discharge or perspiration occurs – indeed, in the eczema/asthma syndrome the homoeopathic remedy, if correct, should first help the asthma, even if the eczema initially becomes worse. Further treatment will then cure the skin manifestations. (This is referred to in Chapter 7 as 'directions of cure'.)

This concept of chronic disease resulting from suppression, particularly of skin ailments, Hahnemann called a miasm, and labelled it Psora (from the itch). Is it not possible that over the years, and even in the present day, we may be contributing to a legacy of chronic disease as a result of some forms of treatment? Certainly, we now see a great deal more chronic illness, arterial and heart disease, arthritis, cancer and psychiatric illness. This may in part be due to our ability to conquer acute diseases, and the fact that people live longer, but are we also contributing to this through pollution of food and atmosphere, and even perhaps by treatment? It is a frightening thought.

Hahnemann's other two miasms were Syphilis and Sycosis, derived mainly from the two venereal diseases, syphilis and gonorrhoea, which were rife in the last century, and which are by no means controlled even with modern therapy. They have also left a legacy of chronic disease affecting not only the genito-urinary system but also joints, arteries, the neurological system and psychiatric illness. They may also have left hereditary traits, causing a wide range of pathological conditions not clearly related to them.

We are now aware that other infections such as diphtheria, measles, scarlet fever, tuberculosis, typhoid fever, malaria, abortus fever and amoebiasis, as well as vaccination, can lead to chronic ill health.

This concept of causal factors in chronic disease is of particular value to the homoeopathic doctor. He has in his Materia Medica remedies specially related to these miasms, which can often assist in helping to cure the patient of his chronic illness.

'Nosodes' are remedies prepared from disease tissue or from cultures of specific organisms, by the process of attenuation and subdivision described in Chapter 6, thus neutralising their toxicity but retaining their ability to antidote and stimulate restorative activity in the tissues of the body.

The treatment of allergies in orthodox medicine is akin to this. Homoeopathic preparations of allergens are available for this purpose and are proving effective.

This description of case-taking may seem a formidable task to the doctor first studying homoeopathy. The whole picture may require to be built up over a number of interviews, and the general practitioner's knowledge of the family and environment will greatly reduce the time spent on actual case-taking. Each doctor will modify his case-taking according to circumstances and as a result of experience, and indeed will evolve his own method. In chronic disease, not easily amenable to other forms of treatment, careful selection of the correct remedy will prove to be justified by the results.

For vivid descriptions of patient types and of the value of observation of a patient's appearance, mannerisms and temperament, the student should read:

*The Patient not the Cure*   Margery G. Blackie
*Homoeopathic Drug Pictures*   Margaret L. Tyler

TABLE 5.1 ACUTE CASE-TAKING SUMMARY

**The Complaint**

Pain, cough, sickness, diarrhoea.

Find out the modalities – what makes it worse or better – movement, pressure, heat, cold, etc.

The character of the cough; the colour and consistency of the sputum, the vomit or the stool.

**Appearance**

Flush, pallor, sweat, delirium.

Rashes.

Appearance of the tongue.

Thirst or absence of thirst.

Fever – its incidence and time aggravation.

**Temperament**

Drowsy, restless, fearful, irritable, desiring attention or to be left alone.

Changes from the normal.

Clinical examination.

TABLE 5.2 CHRONIC CASE-TAKING SUMMARY

**The complaint and present history**

Details of particular symptoms and modalities, and onset.

**Past history**

With particular emphasis on infectious disease, injury, vaccination or failure to recover completely.

**Family history**

Incidence of tuberculosis, cancer, arterial disease, allergy.

**Social history**

Environment, housing, marital relations, smoking, alcohol.

**Physical examination**

Appearance, colouring, manner of patient.

Detailed examination of systems, diagnosis where possible and relevant investigations required.

*continued overleaf*

*Chronic Case-Taking Summary (continued)*

**Homoeopathic history**

*General symptoms*
Reactions to heat, cold, damp, frost, thunder, sea.
Perspiration: parts, character.
Time aggravations.

*Foods* Appetite.
> Strong desires or aversions and foods which disagree: sweet, salt, fat, savouries, spices, eggs, fish, sugar, milk, vinegar.
> Thirst: hot, cold, large, small.

*Sleep* Position in, dreams, better or worse from.

*Menstrual Effects*
a) General upset or improvement before, during or after periods.
b) Particular symptoms of discharge, irritation, etc.

*Mental Symptoms*
These are among the most important in the selection of a homoeopathic remedy.

| | |
|---|---|
| Placid | Sociable |
| Worried | Withdrawn or reticent |
| Irritable | Temper |
| Anticipatory | Sensitive to noise |
| Resentful | Depressed |
| Obstinate | Guilty |
| Rude | Jealous |
| Weepy (relieved or | Loquacious |
| aggravated by sympathy) | Tidiness |

*Fears* Dark | Heights
Alone | Death
Thunder | Illness
Enclosed spaces | Failure
Open spaces | Crowds

*Particular symptoms*
Related to parts or organs. These will have been covered to some extent in the present history. The importance of modalities should be stressed.

| | |
|---|---|
| Head | Stomach |
| Eye | Abdomen |
| Ear | Rectum |
| Nose | Genito-urinary |
| Throat | Back |
| Face | Extremities |
| Mouth | Skin |
| Respiratory | |

## CASE HISTORIES

In order to illustrate the case-taking procedure, I have included a few case histories, not because they are particularly dramatic, although all but two of the patients were helped considerably. They describe the steps in taking the case and the sort of assessment one can make, especially from general and mental symptoms.

It is interesting to note that the three patients with dermatitis each required a different remedy, depending on their general and mental symptoms.

### Case-taking signs
In the case-histories you will come across the signs $>$ and $<$. They indicate the modalities of a symptom, being used in the homoeopathic literature to signify:

> better from or relieved by, $>$
> worse from or aggravated by, $<$.

For example: pain relieved by ($>$) heat, pressure, motion; or pain worse ($<$) from cold, pressure, rest.

On making a prescription, the name of the remedy is followed by the required potency (see Chapter 6) and then by the number of doses; e.g. Lycopodium 30c/3 or Pulsatilla 10M/3.

### *Mrs C., aged 45*

### Complaint
Pain and tightness in her chest for 2 years.
Nervous symptoms.

### Present history
Five years ago had her left breast removed and radiotherapy to follow, causing some fibrosis of her lungs. She was complaining of pain and tightness in her chest for 2 years, worse on walking uphill or on stairs. Also breathless with a sensation of fluttering. Nervous symptoms. Cannot concentrate, upset by the death of her mother two years ago from cancer – she was very attached to her. Had tranquillisers and antidepressants until 6 months ago. Spells when she cannot cope, is tired, irritable and weeps on talking. She is restless, fidgety and depressed in the mornings. Does not want company, and keeps her feelings to herself. Easily startled by noise. Unhappy in her present house.

**Past history**
Appendix removed.

**Family history**
Husband has bronchitis – tends to be depressed.
No family.
Father alive – stays with another daughter.
Mother died of cancer 2 years ago.

**Social history**
Non-smoker. Lives in a council house.

**Homoeopathic history**
*Generals*
< from extremes of heat or cold.
*Sleep:* poor.
*Appetite:* fair.
  *Desires:* plain food, eggs, cheese. Not thirsty.
  *Aversion to:* pickles, fat.
Bowels regular: some spasms of rectal pain and piles.
Urinary frequency.
*Menses:* had X-ray menopause at 40.
Has lost her libido and this worries her for her husband's sake.

*Mentals*
The mental symptoms have been described in the history as they are
  predominant.
She was a dark-haired woman, of medium build. The left breast scar
  was satisfactory and the right breast normal.

With the history of emotional upset over her mother's death, dislike
of company and sympathy, and her tendency to weep and to keep her
feelings in, the remedy Natrum Mur. was indicated.
There were no marked food cravings or weather reactions.
This remedy helped her greatly and was only repeated at two months
and five months interval.

*Mr R. M., aged 26*

**Complaint**
Ulcerative colitis.

**Present history**
Ulcerative colitis for several years. 5 years ago had barium enema and

sigmoidoscopy and attends hospital regularly. Spells of diarrhoea and constipation – now two stools daily with some blood and mucus. No severe pain and weight steady. Anxious to stop drugs. Has had prednisolone enemas and then sulphasalazine 8 daily, now down to 4 daily. Codeine Phos. if loose stools.

**Past history**
Assaulted by a man when 7 years old.
Serious car accident 2 years ago.

**Family history**
Wife alive and well; one boy.
Mother alive and well.
Father had stomach ulcers.

**Social history**
Non-smoker.
Own business as electrician. Was rather unhappy during his college apprenticeship.
A slim man with blue eyes, good colour, scar on his face from car accident. Tongue clean, no abdominal tenderness.

**Homoeopathic history**
*Generals*
Likes heat but worse in a stuffy atmosphere.
Sweaty feet, rather warm.
*Appetite:* good – on high protein, low roughage diet.
 *Desires:* sweet, meat, takes vegetables liquidised, cold milk.
 *Aversion:* curries, much fat.
*Sleep:* normal.

*Mentals*
Shy man, anxious, gets keyed-up on anticipation.
Living in a caravan and altering his house – a bit worried about this.
Occasional temper – not very irritable.
Not weepy or startled. Fairly tidy.
Fear of shut-in places, heights.
If he **has** something on his mind he likes to get it done.

An anxious man with colitis, easily keyed up in anticipation; liking for sweet food.
Lycopodium 30c/3 prescribed.

He continued to have some urging to stool and blood and mucus, and Mercurius Cor. 6x was given twice daily for 2 months, and a further dose of Lycopodium 30 in 4 months' time. In 6 months he was much improved with normal stools, no blood or mucus, and only occasional sulphasalazine. On follow-up a year later he had stopped all medication and was very well.


### *Mrs A., aged 40*

**Complaint**
Migraine for 4 years.


**Present history**
Migraine headaches began when under stress.
She worked for her husband in business, nursed her mother-in-law who
    died, and her own mother who was ill.
Has moved house in the last 2 weeks.
The headaches have been worse in the last 18 months, increasing in
    frequency – now nearly every week and lasting 3–5 days.
Occasionally spots before her eyes. Pain settles above the left eye; she
    has to lie down, and vomits.
She had been investigated: X-ray skull, blood, etc. Only slight anaemia.
She had been on several conventional migraine drugs, which helped her
    attacks to some extent, but tended to upset her. Sometimes she has
    required an injection.


**Past history**
Squint in left eye as a child.
Appendix operation at 36 years.
No known allergies.


**Family History**
Husband alive and well.
Two daughters both well.
Mother alive and well. 72 years.
Father died aged 61 – myocardial infarction.
Twin brother died of leukaemia in 1950.
No family history of migraine.


**Social history**
Lives at home with husband and two daughters.
Not working now.
Non-smoker.

**Homoeopathic history**
*Generals*
Weather no effect.
Damp no effect.
< stuffy room or extreme heat.
Likes fresh air.
Dislikes tight things around her neck.
No perspiration.
*Sleep:* normally good. For a time waking 5 a.m. with palpitations.
*Appetite:* good. Has tried stopping cheese and chocolate for her
    migraine.
    *Desires:* sweet, tasty.
    *Averse:* fat.
    Not thirsty. Likes hot drinks.
Other systems – NAD.
*Menses:* regular, occasional backache the first day.

*Mentals*
Generally placid – used to be upset in anticipation, but less so now.
Shy person, although she is quite sociable, does not go out a lot.
Emotional, weeps easily. Not sure if she likes sympathy.
Shares her worries.
Very tidy.
Fear of heights, and of her headaches.

Pulsatilla was indicated from her dislike of heat and hot places, a
liking for sweet food and her shy emotional personality.

This patient received Pulsatilla 30c/3 with Bryonia to use as an acute
headache remedy, which helped. She steadily improved, resumed a
full-time job and had no further severe headache. Minor headaches
gradually reduced, and she had only one repeat of Pulsatilla six months
after her first dose and has remained well.

*Mrs M., aged 56*

**Complaint**
Huskiness of throat, headache, pressure in sinuses, and post nasal drip.

**Present history**
She is a trained singer and her voice keeps going hoarse. Also nervous
    and weepy since her husband died 5 years ago, weeps every day and
    feels a lump in her throat.
She has had antibiotics and a nasal decongestant with little relief.

**Past history**
From 13–16 years she had diabetes which cleared up with diet.
Disc trouble helped by manipulation.
D and C – fibroids present.

**Family history**
Married twice. Divorced first husband. Second husband died with DLE
and heart attack.
One daughter alive and well – married.

**Social history**
Lives alone. Non-smoker.
Sings with choir and opera chorus.
A thin woman with injected throat. Normal blood pressure.

**Homoeopathic History**
*Generals*
< excessive heat, but also < cold.
Some flushes.
*Appetite:* spells of nervous eating.
  *Desires:* chocolate, savouries.
  *Aversion:* pickles, fat, eggs. Thirsty at times.
Some heartburn, bowels regular.
*Bladder:* up twice at night.
*Menses:* stopped after husband's death 5 years ago.
*Sleep:* good.

*Mentals*
Usually happy but weepy now most days.
Anxious, worries, talks quite a lot.
Good mixer – rather sentimental but says she doesn't expect sympathy.
Affectionate.
Fairly tidy. Sensitive to smells and smoke.
Fear of dying. Noises upset her.

Here we have a lady who has a lot of catarrh and sinus trouble, with
loss of voice. She is nervous and emotional since the death of her
husband, lonely, affectionate and weeps frequently. No very marked
food cravings. Although chilly she dislikes much heat.
    Pulsatilla 10M/3 prescribed.
    Six weeks later she reports feeling much better in every way. Her
breathing is easier, sputum comes up more easily, her headaches are
improved, she is singing clearly and, although still a bit emotional, is
feeling mentally much improved.

*Mrs S., aged 44*

**Complaint**
Ulcerative colitis.

**Present history**
History of ulcerative colitis for 3 years. Had been in hospital 1½ years ago, when the condition was diagnosed. She was on sulphasalazine and prednisolone enemas, improved for 6 months and then relapsed, with loss of weight and depression. 3 months ago she had more bleeding and last month was on prednisolone 10mg daily and steroid enemas. She was anxious to try homoeopathy to see if she could reduce her medication.

**Past history**
Tendency to diarrhoea if upset.
6 years ago a spell of weakness of her right arm and leg thought to be
   possible MS. Steroids given and improved. Still a little weakness.

**Family history**
Husband had tuberculosis – a lot of worry over him.

**Homoeopathic history**
*Generals*
Chilly person but with hot hands and feet in bed.
Sweat of feet and hands.
*Appetite –*
   *Desires:* savouries, eggs.
   *Aversion:* fat, salt, sauces.
*Menses:* regular.

*Mentals*
Sociable person, weepy, sympathetic, better from consolation.
Untidy, startled easily, worries, gets keyed up.
Fear thunder.
Nightmares of death.

   A sensitive outgoing person, untidy, emotional, better from consolation with fear of thunder and dreams. Chilly, liking for savouries,
thirsty for cold drink. History of colitis with bleeding.
   This picture suggested Phosphorus, which was prescribed in 30c
potency, 3 doses.
   Steady improvement after this, gradual reduction of cortisone which
was stopped in 3 months.

Phosphorus repeated after 8 months. 2 years later slight recurrence after an antibiotic for a throat infection. Gaertner 30c/3 given, the related bowel nosode.

Reports 3 years later – no further relapse, very well, no medication.

*Mr R., aged 42*

**Complaint**

This man, who was an engineer and worked with synthetic oils, came complaining of a rash on his hands and feet for 4 months following a domestic upset. He had also been off work for 9 months,

His palms and soles were covered with small itchy blisters which burst and wept moisture.

He had been using steroid creams and taking diazepam.

**Past history**
Nil.

**Family history**
Wife under psychiatric care – she had been running up debts.
One daughter.

**Social history**
Smokes 40 per day. Drinks some beer. Plays tennis and badminton.

**Homoeopathic history**
*Generals*
$>$ heat. $<$ cold.
*Appetite:* good.
   *Desires–pickles, salt,* sweet, some fat, cheese, eggs.
*Sleep:* good.
Other systems: nil.

*Mentals*
*Worries.*
Irritable – slow to reach a temper.
A bit self-conscious, upset in anticipation.
*Tidy* and *exact.*
Likes to be busy, frustrated at being off work.
Can be a bit emotional.
A tall grey-haired man.

A chilly patient, with liking for tasty, salty foods, tidy in his habits, but irritable and frustrated.

Nux Vomica 30c was prescribed.

Within 10 days his feet were improved and his palms less moist and not so itchy. He was keen to get back to work.

Within a month his hands were almost clear and he had started a clerical job.

## *Mrs E., aged 60*

**History**

Dry, cracked skin lesions on both hands and wrists, and spots on her back for several years.

Catarrh, blocked nose, loss of smell.

Nervous, excitable and weepy.

Nursed her mother-in-law for 8 years – she died last year and she misses her. She also misses her job as a theatre nurse.

**Past history**

Catarrh, and wheezing after being in the USA.

**Family history**

Husband alive and well.

Two children both married – high blood pressure during second pregnancy.

Mother had thyroid operation – died of pneumonia at 81.

Father died of a stroke at 79.

**Social history**

Lives with her husband.

Smokes 20 per day.

**Homoeopathic history**

*Generals*

< heat. > cold.

*Appetite:* good

    *Desires* – savouries, *salt*.

    *Aversion* – sweet, pickles, fat.

Thirst for water and coffee.

Bowels regular.

Catarrh and wheezing.

Back trouble with a disc – now improved.

*Menses:* stopped at 52.

*Sleep:* wakes early – difficulty rising.

*Mentals*
Nervous, easily startled, upset in anticipation.
*Weepy* – upset by sympathy.
Used to like people but cannot now be bothered going to the shops.
Not irritable, but rather restless and impatient.
Average tidy. No fears.
Although she nursed her mother-in-law for years she found her very
   demanding, and was resentful about this, though less so now.

A fair, plump rather overweight lady with a slight tremor. No thyroid
enlargement.
   BP 220/115.
   Dry eruption on hands, wrists and back, thickened nails.
   With the history of some resentment, nervousness, startled by noise,
weepy but upset by sympathy, together with < heat, desire for salt and
a skin eruption probably of nervous origin, Natrum Mur. 30c was
prescribed.
   This remedy helped her emotionally, her BP came down to 170/90
over the next few months and her hands healed completely in three
months. She has received some other remedies for rheumatism and
other complaints, but her hands remained healed.

## *P., aged 16*

**Complaint**
This young man presented with a moist itchy eruption on his hands, of 3
years duration. Two years previously his mother had left the family and
his skin became worse. He had used a steroid ointment with only
temporary effect.

**Past history**
Leg operation.
Some history of asthma – allergy to cats, strawberries and oil.

**Homoeopathic history**
*Generals*
Prefers some heat but no marked heat, cold or weather aggravations.
*Appetite:* good.
   *Desires* – most foods, sweet, fat, milk.
Bowels normal.
Sleep good.

*Mentals*
A good mixer, tendency to worry, a bit emotional, fear of the dark.
Not irritable.
Rather untidy. Artistic, fond of painting.

On the basis of the skin lesion, liking for fat and sweet food, and sociable, untidy temperament, he was prescribed Sulphur 12c and then 30c.

His skin cleared up after the first prescription, and a slight relapse two months later responded to the 30c potency.

## *Mark, aged 3¾*

A typical child seen at outpatients is the boy with recurring coughs and colds.

He had had repeated coughs and colds since he was a baby, seven times each winter. He developed a head cold then a cough, dry and sore, then fever, and usually had to receive antibiotics so often that his doctor and his mother were concerned.

**Past history**
No eczema or other illness.

**Family history**
Nil.
A fair haired boy, with big pupils.

**Homoeopathic history**
*Generals*
Warm person.
*Appetite. Desires* – sweet, cheese, salt, sauce, butter.
Thirst for water.

*Mentals*
A sociable, rather wild boy with tempers.

A hot, sociable child with thirst and liking for tasty food, sweet and butter, suggested Sulphur. This was prescribed in 30c potency.

Following this, his health greatly improved and his colds and coughs disappeared.

*G., girl, aged 7*

**Complaint and present history**

Bronchitis every 6 weeks for the last 9 months, the last attack being 2 weeks ago. Numerous antibiotics.

**Past history**

Wheeze off and on since 9 months of age.

2 years ago acute asthma – seen at Allergy Clinic and found to be sensitive to grass, pollens and house dust, but not to animals. Injections given with slight benefit.

Attacks start as a cold, then sneezing, sore throat, wheeze and then cough with green sputum. No change at the sea.

Measles at 3 years.

**Family history**

Mother and father well.

Grandfather had asthma.

A fair, slim girl with long eyelashes and dark blue eyes.

Small tonsils, no glands. Chest clear on examination.

**Homoeopathic history**

*Generals*

Upset by heat; sweat of neck and feet.

*Appetite. Desires* – onions, cheese, eggs. Quite thirsty for cold milk or water.

*Mentals*

Well behaved girl, shy but makes friends.

Affectionate. Weepy when ill.

A bit stubborn, not anxious.

The picture presenting here is like Phosphorus or Pulsatilla, but in view of the fact that she was upset by heat and rather weepy, Pulsatilla 30 was given.

Six weeks later mother reports that she coughed up a lot of yellow catarrh after the remedy and has then been very well. She is eating well and has had no further wheeze.

Apart from obviously incurable conditions, where the most one can expect is palliation and some relief of symptoms, there are some patients who seem to fail to respond to any form of treatment, a large group being the neurotic patients whose symptoms constantly change. There are also some patients who fail to improve with homoeopathic remedies, in spite of reasonably clear prescribing symptoms. Some may genuinely fail to react to homoeopathy. In some the doctor's failure to select the correct remedy or potency, or to extract the really relevant symptoms, may lead to disappointing results. The art of questioning and weighing up the relevance of symptoms is a very skilled one. Some physicians seem to have an intuitive gift for this.

Below are two case histories where seemingly indicated remedies failed to act. This experience should not make the doctor give up. He should be spurred to read more widely, to re-study the case, and even take it afresh.

### *Miss D., aged 43*

**Complaint**
Diarrhoea in spells of two or three days every 3 weeks since the age of 16 years.

**History**
Periodic bouts of colicky pain followed by loose stools and burning yellow mucus lasting a few days every 2–3 weeks. Also epigastric pain with heartburn and acid risings, usually relieved by eating and worse when empty, better from warm drinks. Worse before her menses. Sinusitis and occasional migraine. Barium meal 10 years ago showed some duodenal irritation, but barium enema was negative. Treated with propantheline bromide, antacids, chlordiazepoxide. Tends to be travel sick.

**Past history**
Pulmonary tuberculosis and cavity 23 years ago, with phrenic crush and chemotherapy.
A laparotomy 18 years ago – appendix removed but no evidence of abdominal tuberculosis.

**Family history**
Mother arthritic, 83.
Father 92, in psychogeriatric hospital.
Two brothers died, one of tuberculosis.

**Social history**
Lives with her parents.
Works as a nursing sister.
Non-smoker.

**Homoeopathic symptoms**
*Generals*
Better from heat, used to feel cold, hands and feet cold.
Stomach: poor appetite. Desires tasty food but upset by fried food, rich, sweet, fruit.
Sleep: good. Vivid dreams.
Nose: sinusitis, green catarrh.
Menses: regular but scanty, dysmenorrhoea quite bad before and during first 2 days of period.

*Mentals*
Sociable. Better from company, likes affection.
A bit irritable.
Not very worried or anxious.
Sensitive but does not actually weep much.
No fears.
Rather tidy. Fond of music.
She does not admit to any particular stress, apart from those in her work, and her old father. She has had no unhappy love affair and does not appear very anxious.
A barium enema shows a rather smooth descending colon with lack of haustral markings. No evidence of neoplasm. Barium meal and follow through showed a partial volvulus of the stomach but no other abnormality in duodenum or small bowel.
Over the past 15 months this lady has attended regularly at monthly intervals and received a number of remedies. At times she seemed a little better, and she now looks well with no loss of weight but still has epigastric pain and bouts of colic with burning yellow stools for 2–3 days every 3 weeks.

**Remedies given**
Tuberculinum Bov., Graphites, Gaertner, Phosphorus, Sulphur, Nux Vom., Aloes in 30c potencies, and also low potencies of Podophyllum and Mercurius Cor. and Colocynth for colic.
One feels that there must be a suitable remedy to cure this patient. She has also had bran, and a spell off milk and wheat.


*C., boy, aged 8*


**Complaint**
Psoriasis since the age of 3 years.

**Present history**
Psoriasis began in the scrotal region and spread to cover large areas of

the body, arms, legs, scalp and above the ears. Large scaly plaques, itchy and dry; scalp has a thick scale. He has been in hospital and had extensive local applications, mainly of steroid ointments which help temporarily. It usually improves at the sea and in the sun. Was aggravated after chickenpox.

**Past history**
Measles, chickenpox, mumps. Inoculations with triple vaccine and polio
  – no upset.
Pneumonia at 2 years.
Tonsils removed at 6 years.

**Family history**
Mother: has migraine.
Father: well.
Two brothers and one sister well.
Two of his uncles had psoriasis.

**Social history**
Family middle class, no financial problems. Father seems rather over-powering and intense.
A dark, slim boy, with blocked nose and warts on his hands.

**Homoeopathic history**
*Generals*
Warm child. Sweat of head and feet.
*Appetite:* good – eats a lot but remains thin.
   *Desires:* – sweet, tasty foods, sauce, eggs, milk, salt.
   *Aversions* – fat.
Bowels regular.

*Mentals*
Sociable, bright boy; likes older people.
Not very demonstrative; some tempers; easily bored.
At one time destructive and talkative at school.
No fears, not very tidy, not weepy.
Likes change and new things.

**Remedies given**
Tuberculinum 30c caused slight improvement and his warts rapidly
  disappeared.
His skin seemed to improve quite a lot, especially his legs, after Sulphur
  and Phosphorus. Marked improvement after Morgan Co. 30c.
His nose remained very blocked and Bacillinum and Thuja were given
  with no effect. The scalp remained bad and Sulphur and then Mor-

gan Co. were repeated, and Graphites all in 30c potency, single doses at monthly intervals. The skin then began to get steadily worse and he had a further spell in hospital.

He became depressed, difficult at school, restless and rebellious. Medorrhinum, Sulphur and Staphisagria were tried. He then went to Israel to a special clinic with bathing in the Dead Sea, and rubbing the scalp with salt, and this improved him a bit; on returning, in view of the improvement with salt, Natrum Mur. was given. He is happier but the skin remains a problem.

Skin conditions which are better at the sea often respond well to Medorrhinum but this remedy did not help. Perhaps the remedies were changed too often, even although 4–6 weeks elapsed between each. Perhaps the potencies were wrong.

One has seen cases of psoriasis which are markedly improved by homoeopathy and some actually cured. In other patients seemingly indicated remedies fail to act at all. A puzzling illness!

# Chapter 6

# The Preparation of Homoeopathic Remedies

Homoeopathic remedies can be prepared from any substance which has either a toxic effect on the body or which exerts a chemical change on it. Remedies are prepared from plant tinctures, salts, metals, snake and spider venoms and even synthetic drugs.

The technique used by the homoeopathic pharmacist is laid down with great accuracy in Hahnemann's *Materia Medica Pura* and also in his volume on *Chronic Diseases*.

The standard pharmaceutical texts are: *The American Homoeopathic Pharmacopoeia* 1928, *The British Pharmacopoeia* 1882, and J. H. Clarke's *Dictionary of Materia Medica*.

In the case of insoluble substances, one part of the mother substance and nine or ninety-nine parts of an inert medium, namely coarse lactose, are triturated (ground) with mortar and pestle, usually in three separate quantities. One part of this is again triturated with nine or ninety-nine parts lactose. After three stages of trituration this material can be suspended in a fluid medium, and thereafter the technique is the same as that described below for tinctures.

Homoeopathic remedies can be used in mother tincture, diluted for either local or oral medication, or they can be prepared by the technique of serial dilution and succussion, or mechanical shock. These solutions are known as 'potencies' because of the apparent increase in their clinical effect with increasing stages of preparation.

There are two ranges of potency. The decimal scale 1 in 10 are designated 'x' or 'D' potencies, and the centesimal scale 1 in 100 are called 'c' potencies. In the United Kingdom a potency written omitting the letter 'c' is taken to be a centesimal potency. The reader will find both usages, in this book as well as in the literature generally. An additional range of very high potencies, called 'M' potencies, are diluted 1 in a 1000 parts between succussions, and are largely made in the USA.

The extracted mother tincture of the fresh growing plant is diluted in 40 per cent alcohol in the above two dilutions, one drop to nine or ninety-nine drops of diluent. The liquid is shaken ten times in a sealed vial, two-third filled (i.e. by the process known as succussion). Using a separate pipette and vial at each stage, one drop of this solution is again diluted and succussed. It is important to realise that the homoeopathic potency is not simply a highly diluted solution, but one made by this rigid procedure of serial dilution and succussion.

It is now thought that this technique may alter the physical state of the solution in such a way that the specificity of the original substance is maintained, even at high degrees of potentisation. It is probable, by the laws of physical chemistry, that a potency of 12c or higher will not actually contain a single molecule of the original substance; but in practice these high potencies do seem to be active.

Only certain stages of potency are used in clinical practice, the commonest being 1x, 3x, 6x, 12x, 6c, 12c, 30c, 200c, 1M (or 1000c), 10M, 50M and CM.

The remedies are available in tinctures, tablets or granules. Granules are prepared with 100 per cent sucrose as a base, inoculated with the required liquid potency. Tablets contain 20 per cent sucrose in lactose as a base.

Homoeopathic remedies are available in the United Kingdom on NHS prescription, but should always be obtained from a reputable manufacturing homoeopathic chemist. The manufacturer will supply details of the preparations, which can be issued to local chemists.

# Chapter 7

# Principles of Prescribing, and Administration of the Remedy

TABLE 7.1    PRINCIPLES OF HOMOEOPATHIC PRESCRIBING
The Like Remedy
The Single Remedy
The Single Dose (in potentised form)
Homoeopathic Aggravation
Directions of Cure

## THE LIKE REMEDY

Two things are necessary for the successful selection of the similar remedy: a clear picture of the patient's symptoms and a comprehensive knowledge of the Materia Medica.

It has been stressed already that the symptoms characteristic of the patient as an individual, in his reaction to the causative factors in his illness, play the most important part in building up the symptom picture.

The modalities of the particular symptoms are essential in their evaluation. Above all, the whole patient must be assessed, including his physical features, general reactions and emotional and temperamental attributes.

Having obtained a full picture of the patient we must now seek in the Materia Medica a remedy which has, as nearly as possible, a similar picture in its provings and toxicology. The importance of the mental and general symptoms of the patient should also rank high in the remedy picture if a correct selection is to be made.

Different doctors have their own method of selecting a suitable remedy. With a good knowledge of Materia Medica it may be possible to see the indicated remedy clearly after taking the case, without the aid of books. It is wise to list the main symptoms with their modalities, and to note any strange, rare or peculiar symptoms. Then one should look at the patient as a whole, as described under 'case-taking', noting the appearance, and the general and mental symptoms.

Select from them the symptoms which you cannot omit because they are so marked. Then take one of the repertories mentioned in Chapter 4, Kent's being the most commonly used, and see what remedies cover most of the listed symptoms. Next look again at the Materia Medica of these few remedies to decide on your choice. You can give points, 3, 2 or 1 to particular remedies, depending on the weight of the type in the repertory and then add up the score, selecting the one with most points.

Mention has been made of using remedies known to have particular value in relation to organs and systems. Section II may prove helpful in this respect.

You will find that there are considerable differences of opinion among homoeopathic doctors on whether or when to use high or low potencies. This is a matter for individual choice and experience. I have tried to give the broad consensus view of this aspect of prescribing, but good results are obtained with either method.

## THE SINGLE REMEDY

The concept that the remedy acts as a stimulus to the tissues of the body, and that its selection is based on the Materia Medica picture, supports the view that wherever possible a single homoeopathic remedy should be prescribed. Occasionally a high potency of one remedy is given, followed by a low potency of a remedy with more local tissue affinity. This is discussed more fully under 'Administration of the Remedy' (page 56).

The single remedy method of prescribing is based on the views of Hahnemann and Kent (of America) and is the one mainly used in the British Isles, in the USA, and in South America. In many other countries, and notably in France and Germany, a system of poly-pharmacy is used by many doctors and lay practitioners. With this method, several remedies are combined in the one preparation and are prescribed mainly on pathological indications, apparently with considerable success.

## THE SINGLE DOSE

Again, the concept that the remedy acts as a 'trigger effect' to the body's natural reaction points to the necessity for a single dose, the minimum stimulus required. In chronic disease this is usually given as a single powder, or three powders 4 hourly, the single divided dose of a high potency: 30c or 10M. The effect of this dose may last for some weeks, and even occasionally for 2–3 months. *As long as improvement is continuing no further dose should be given.*

In acute illness the stimulus of this dose will be rapidly used up and a further dose will be necessary, the speed of repetition depending on the acuteness of the condition, usually at 2 hourly intervals to begin with and then 4 hourly. In a very acute state a remedy like Carbo Veg. or Arsenicum Album may be required every 5 minutes.

## THE HOMOEOPATHIC AGGRAVATION

Because the remedy causes the patient to react, it may result in some initial aggravation of symptoms, e.g. a skin lesion may become more irritable, coryza or wheezing may get worse. This is not always a bad thing as it means that the patient is reacting, and after the first week in a chronic disease improvement will usually follow. This aggravation is seldom seen in acute illness, and only in some chronic cases. It is usually not very severe, but may cause some concern, for example, where a child's eczema seems initially to be getting worse. An explanation to the parent or patient that this will soon subside is usually all that is required. It is important, therefore, in chronic cases not to see the patient too often, or the doctor may be tempted to change the remedy instead of allowing the aggravation to subside and improvement to start.

Non-interference with remedy action should be stressed again, as long as improvement is occurring.

## DIRECTIONS OF CURE

An interesting observation in medicine in general, but in homoeopathy in particular, is the fact that if a remedy is curing the patient, symptoms and signs will progress in a particular direction.

> From within outwards.
> From above downwards.
> From more important to less important organs.
> In the reverse order of their development.

The eczema/asthma syndrome is a good case in point. Asthma is the more important and inner affection, and in curing this the eczema may get a bit worse at first – which is the correct direction of cure.

Occasionally a patient with a severe chest or gastric disorder who is improving may notice the recurrence of a skin lesion or discharging ear, apparently 'cured' many years before. Perhaps it was merely suppressed and the more serious ailment developed. Now it is recurring, and it too will eventually be cured. (See also Chapter 5.)

## ADMINISTRATION OF THE REMEDY

As already stated in Chapter 6, these are available as tinctures, granules or tablets.

### Tinctures
Tinctures may be applied locally as a solution, usually 10 drops to half a pint of water, e.g. Calendula lotion for wounds and cuts, Arnica lotion for bruises. A number of ointments are also available for local application. (See Chapter 9 on injuries and accidents.) Tinctures are sometimes given orally as drops, e.g. 5 drops three times daily of Crataegus, Iberis or Convallaria in heart conditions.

Low potency solutions of 1x or 3x are available for oral use, e.g. Hydrastis, Kali Bich. or Pulsatilla for catarrhal states.

### Tablets
Both high and low potencies are available as tablets. Most low potencies, such as 1x, 3x and 6x are given in this form, one tablet two or three times daily over periods of some weeks. These are often prescriptions for local tissues or organs, e.g. Sulphur for the itch of skin lesions, Carbo Sulph. for venous stasis and congestion, Hamamelis in venous thrombosis. These low potencies can also be given in acute conditions, repeated every 2 hours, and first aid kits often contain such tablets for colds, coughs, injuries and early fevers.

### Granules
Some doctors use granules, made up in small paper packets or powders. Less than a salt-spoonful is necessary for each dose, only a few granules having the desired effect, when placed in the mouth or below the tongue. The exact quantity is not important but the intervals of repetition are. The same dose can be given to infants, adults or the very old. Most potencies from the lowest to the highest are available in this form.

## Manufacturers' packs

These are specially prepared and sealed, and can be delivered direct to the patient, either on EC.10 or privately, or can be stocked by your local chemist for issue to your patients. Each pack contains two bottles, one with liquid, the other with tablets, and is available for all common remedies in a variety of potencies.

## What potency do I prescribe, and when?

The potency most commonly used in the United Kingdom is the 30c, for both acute and chronic illness. High potencies, 30c, 200c, 1M and 10M are used in cases of acute illness and in patients with strong mental symptoms in their case picture. They may also be used in deep-seated chronic illness.

Mention has been made of the use of tinctures and low potencies already. They are most useful as local organ or tissue remedies, although some doctors prescribe low potencies in every case. They are also of value for prolonged use when there is severe pathological change, e.g. Bryonia or Rhus Tox. 6x in chronic arthritis. These low potencies are in small but material doses.

In *acute disease* the remedy stimulus must be repeated frequently, as already stated, and a powder or tablet may be given every 2 or 4 hours, or in very acute states every 5 minutes. When prescribing in the home this can best be done by giving one powder or tablet dry, and dissolving one in half a cup or glass of cold water. The solution is stirred and a teaspoonful given every 2–4 hours. After the remedy is finished the cup and spoon should be thoroughly washed and scalded, or put in a hot oven, before being used again. If the remedy is changed during an illness it is wise to use a fresh cup and spoon.

The reason for scalding or dry heating a cup or spoon or a medicine glass is to ensure removal of potency from the glass, and was recommended as a result of laboratory experiments by the late W. E. Boyd of Glasgow. It is unlikely that a potency leached into glass would affect another person drinking from that glass; but potency energy is so little understood that it is possible that another remedy added to the same glass without adequate cleaning could become contaminated, and thus fail to act.

It should be stated again that half a salt-spoonful of granules or one tablet is adequate for each dose; repetition is what increases the effect in acute illness, not the size of each dose. A 30c or 10M potency is usually given; and the *same* dose and potency can be given to an infant, a grown man or an elderly lady. In acute situations it may be necessary to change the remedy if a response is not seen within a few hours, or certainly the following day. The correct homoeopathic remedy acts very quickly. Carbo. Veg. or Arsenicum Album should show an effect within 5–10 minutes, and remedies in pneumonia or tonsillitis will help as fast as an antibiotic, if selected accurately.

In *chronic disease* a single or divided single dose should be given as already mentioned.

This should be allowed to act as long as improvement is taking place, particularly if the patient feels better in himself, even although the local symptoms have not yet cleared up entirely. If relapse occurs with the same symptoms, a repeat dose is called for, either of the same potency or the next higher potency. If there is no improvement after 2–3 weeks, or the symptom picture has changed, a different or related remedy may be required.

**The second prescription**
When a patient returns for his second visit the doctor must attempt to assess any progress. This requires experience, as well as the ability to judge critically what the patient tells you about any aggravation, initially or continuing, and any improvement. Is the improvement in a local symptom, or in his general well-being or mental and emotional state? The latter are often more important than a purely local improvement in a pain or swelling, even though this may be the patient's main complaint. There are some patients who quickly say they are better, to please the doctor; others are very reluctant to admit any change, but on questioning are found to have considerable improvement in certain aspects of their health. Do not accept the first 'I am better' or 'I am no better' immediately. Go back through your list of symptoms from the first interview, with their modalities, and find out whether they are different or better, and in what way. In particular try to assess whether the patient is 'better in himself'.

The choices open to you are to leave the remedy to continue acting, and if you feel it necessary, to give placebo; to repeat the same remedy in the same potency; to change the potency; or to select a new remedy on the symptoms *now* presenting. A graphical way of assessing your last prescription and deciding on the next is given in Table 7.2.

TABLE 7.2    DEDUCTIONS FROM EFFECTS OF THE REMEDY

1.  *No change*

      May mean           a)  remedy wrong
                           b)  potency wrong
                           c)  patient sluggish in reacting
                           d)  slow-acting remedy

      Reassess.

2  *Steady rapid improvement, without any aggravation*

      This means          a)  remedy and potency exactly correspond
                           b)  or disease not deeply rooted

steady
improvement

no
aggravation

      No further remedy.

3.  *Sharp aggravation, then quick improvement;*
    *the improvement being long lasting*

      This means          a)  remedy correct
                           b)  reaction vigorous
                           c)  no tendency to structural changes
                           d)  good prognosis

steady
improvement,
even for months

short
aggravation

      Patients usually do best who get this homoeopathic aggravation.
      No further remedy – allow action to continue.

**4.**  *Long aggravation with slow improvement*

Means case almost incurable, vitality being low.

long
aggravation

slow
improvement

Do not repeat too soon – wait till patient has sufficient strength to react to another dose.

**5.**  *Long aggravation with slow decline of patient*

Means incurable case, or potency too high for feeble reaction of patient.

long
aggravation

slow decline

Incurable is only used in homoeopathic sense of the term – you can alleviate greatly.

**6.**  *An aggravation followed by return of old symptoms, in reverse order of their appearing*

This is the best we can desire – *and the doctor must not interfere.*
These old symptoms usually disappear in a short time – if some of them persist, they rank high in next prescription.

## PRECAUTIONS WHEN USING HOMOEOPATHIC REMEDIES

A great many rigid rules were laid down in the past, regarding what patients should or should not do when taking remedies. Some of these perhaps go to unnecessary extremes, but certain suggestions may be helpful.

The remedy should be taken when the mouth is clean and not contaminated by food, drink, tobacco, peppermint or strong toothpaste.

As far as possible, other drugs should not be taken along with homoeopathic remedies, although in certain situations this is unavoidable. Large amounts of coffee and tea can be classed as drugs.

Remedies should not be exposed to strong sunlight, and should be kept away from strong odours, e.g. camphor, which is included in many proprietary inhalants or 'rubs', mothballs, menthol, and eucalyptus. Patients should preferably avoid these things while taking their remedy, as they may interfere with its action.

# Chapter 8

# *Research*

## SCIENTIFIC EVIDENCE OF HOMOEOPATHIC PRINCIPLES

There are two fundamental principles underlying the practice of homoeopathic medicine. Both have already been mentioned.

1 The Simile Principle
2 The Activity of Potentised Preparations

The idea and use of the simile principle did not originate with Hahnemann or with the introduction of clinical homoeopathy. It can be traced back through history, even to the time of Hippocrates. A review of this can be found in Linn J. Boyd's book *The Simile in Medicine.*

Coming nearer to the present day, I have already mentioned that we may well be using the homoeopathic principle in conventional medicine without being aware of it, whenever we treat a patient with something which is also known to cause similar symptoms. The use of an identical substance, in potency, to that which caused the symptoms, may more accurately be described as 'isopathy', for example a potency of penicillin to clear up the allergic rash caused by penicillin. This has been demonstrated in a wide range of allergic conditions, but is still a kind of simile action. The use of vaccines and desensitising agents also comes within this definition. The recent research and clinical trial of injection of cells or tissue products taken from a patient or animal into that same subject, after modification, is almost identical to the use of homoeopathic nosodes, e.g. treatment of Burkitt's lymphoma, and recent studies on the leukaemia of cats.

Homoeopathic doctors have been potentising tissue and discharges from patients with measles, tuberculosis, diphtheria and septic lesions for many years, and using these remedies to treat patients. It is usually done when the patient 'has never felt well since' an illness, or has residual damage from it, rather than as a direct treatment in the acute situation.

Immunological research has developed widely in the last few years, demonstrating the importance of the reaction of the patient's own cells and antibodies to outside stimuli, or even to those within himself, varying from individual to individual. The importance of the patient's reaction, and the variations of response in individuals, has always been a fundamental of the homoeopathic physician's approach to a clinical problem.

## CLINICAL TRIALS

Can homoeopathy be proved by clinical trials? We are always accused of failing to produce double blind statistics of clinical results, but are these anyway as reliable as some would have us believe? Are control cases really identical to those receiving medication, in terms of age, sex, build, temperament or individual sensitivity? Many drugs are tested for their short-term relief of local symptoms, without any evidence that they cure the patient.

The double blind technique is not easily adapted to homoeopathic prescribing, for several reasons. Only rarely does a homoeopathic physician prescribe one remedy for a specific illness, even a sore throat or pneumonia. The remedy must be selected for the individual, even though the bacteriology may be the same.

In trials of antirheumatic drugs or analgesics, the effects are assessed on the relief of symptoms over a short period, comparing this with another drug or a placebo, in a crossover trial. In a homoeopathic prescription, the relief of pain is not necessarily the criterion of successful cure. The patient's whole well-being, his emotional reactions as well as local symptoms, must be assessed in deciding the effectiveness of a remedy. However, a recent trial conducted by Dr R. Gibson et al.[1,2] has demonstrated that homoeopathic remedies, selected on an individual basis, and compared in one series to aspirin, and in another to placebo, using a double blind technique, do show a definite clinical effect. The usual parameters for assessing response in rheumatoid arthritis were used, and in a good percentage of patients other forms of therapy were stopped or reduced, while the patients showed significant clinical improvement.

Paterson[3] demonstrated the effects of a potency of mustard gas given prophylactically, as well as after application of the liquid gas, to volunteers in a double blind controlled trial in 1943.

Arnica has long been used in homoeopathy for treating injury, bruises and the effects of damage in cerebrovascular or coronary artery disease. Clinical trials of Arnica in these situations are being carried out, so far with limited success, but again with the difficulty of using a single remedy for a number of patients, some of whom would respond better to a selected individual remedy, depending on their clinical symptoms.[4,5,6]

A trial on the use of homoeopathic potencies of house dust in cases of allergy is proceeding at present.

A clinical double blind trial using Cantharis potency in cases of acute cystitis is also being carried out throughout Britain.

## PROVINGS

Mention has been made of the technique of 'proving' remedies by giving repeated doses to healthy volunteers, and thus provoking symptoms, which go to form the 'drug pictures' of the Materia Medica. While this is valuable for obtaining data about new substances which could be used in treatment, the technique of 'proving' is also a form of trial, as the doses given are often in potency form as high as 30c or 200c. Controls are included using placebo, and the crossover method also is frequently used. These provings are themselves demonstrations of potency action, and have been recorded over many years in the *British Homoeopathic Journal* and in foreign journals. They are continuing with even more rigid control at the Royal London Homoeopathic Hospital.

## LABORATORY EVIDENCE OF ACTIVITY OF HOMOEOPATHIC POTENCIES

While it is now accepted that measurable effects can be recorded up to dilutions of $10^{-15}$, this in homoeopathic terms is no more than a potency of 8c. Ian A. Boyd[7] has demonstrated the clear effects of perfusion of $10^{-19}$g/ml acetylcholine on sensitised frog hearts. However, homoeopathic physicians frequently use far greater dilutions in their potencies, with apparent clinical effects. It should be reiterated that a potency of 30c is not merely a dilution of $10^{-60}$, but a preparation resulting from serial dilution in stages of $\frac{1}{100} \times 30$, with succussion or mechanical shock between each stage. It is this serial dilution with succussion which we believe to be vital in the production of a potency, which may not act on a material level at all, but by means of some energy source preserved in the solvent. Theories about this have been discussed by Barnard[8] and others.

Although no satisfactory explanation of potency action is as yet available, many experiments performed in laboratory situations demonstrate that these potencies do have an action recordable by present-day techniques. I have selected a few of these which are well documented, and convincing.

W. E. Boyd[9] (Glasgow 1954) published a paper demonstrating the effects of 30c potencies of mercuric chloride on a starch-diastase preparation, and also experiments on frog heart preparations. This paper shows overwhelming statistical evidence of activity at 30c potency.

E. Heintz[10, 11] (1958, 1964, 1970, 1973) demonstrated effects of potencies up to 18x on the behaviour of fish under controlled conditions.

Boiron and Zervudacki[12] (1963, 1967) studied the effects of potencies of disodium hydrogen arsenate (3x–19x) on the respiration of wheat coleoptiles.

Netien, Boiron et al.[13] (1966) carried out a series of experiments to demonstrate the effect of potencies of copper sulphate (15c) on plants poisoned by copper sulphate.

Cier et al.[14, 15] (1965, 1967) published papers demonstrating the influence of preliminary treatment with Alloxan (9c potency) on the diabetogenic action of Alloxan on mice, and also its use after injections of Alloxan. This is an interesting paper.

Boiron[16] (1973) describes the action of dilutions of 5c, 7c and 15c of copper sulphate on the respiration of Salvinia Natans.

Aubin et al.[17] (1976) show the action of dilutions of Arnica on the dehydrogenase levels in the muscles of experimental rats undergoing exercise.

M. C. Boffa[18, 19, 20] (1973, 1976) carried out some interesting experiments with the venom of Naja Nigricollis, a remedy used in homoeopathic practice.

Aubin and Bildet[21] (1979) have studied the effect of intraperitoneal injections of Phosphorus 7c and 15c on the liver enzymes of rats poisoned by carbon tetrachloride.

Moss (from the Physiology Department, Glasgow University) has been studying the effects of potencies of homoeopathic remedies on the movement of macrophages in guinea pigs, and leucocytes in patients with inflammatory conditions, in controlled laboratory studies. These experiments have produced some very significant effects, compared to controls, but as yet only in isolated cases. They justify further repeated experiments.

Research departments, particularly in France and Germany, are continuing to produce experimental evidence of potency action, but what is really required in the United Kingdom is a determined effort by several laboratories with trained expert personnel and financial support to find out what happens when solutions are serially diluted and succussed, and to demonstrate clearly that activity of some kind is present in these solutions.

Clinicians using homoeopathy have no doubt whatever that their remedies have an action other than placebo effect in their patients. Somehow this must be investigated further, not just for the sake of homoeopathy, but also because the phenomenon of the potentised solution could have repercussions on many fields of medicine, physiology and physics.

# REFERENCES

1. Gibson, R. G., Gibson, S. L. M., MacNeill, A. D., Gray, G. H., Carson Dick, W. and Watson Buchanan, W. Salicylates and homoeopathy in rheumatoid arthritis: Preliminary observations. *Brit. J. clin. Pharmac.* 1978, **6**, 391.
2. Gibson, R. G., Gibson, S. L. M., MacNeill, A. D. and Watson Buchanan, W. Homoeopathic therapy in rheumatoid arthritis: Evaluation by double-blind clinical therapeutic trial. *Brit. J. clin. Pharmac.* 1980, **9**, 453–9.
3. Paterson, J. Report on mustard gas experiments (Glasgow and London). *Brit. Hom. J.,* 1943, January 25th. Reviews by Kennedy, C. O. *Brit. Hom. J.* 1973, **62**, 233.
4. Campbell, Anthony. Two pilot controlled trials of Arnica Montana. *Brit. Hom. J.* 1976, **65**, 154.
5. Savage, R. H. and Roe, P. F. A double blind trial to assess the benefit of Arnica Montana in acute stroke illness. *Brit. Hom. J.* 1977, **66**, 207.
6. Savage, R. H. and Roe, P. F. A further double blind trial to assess the benefit of Arnica Montana in acute stroke illness. *Brit. Hom. J.* 1978, **67**, 210.
7. Boyd, I. A. Homoeopathy through the eyes of a physiologist. *Brit. Hom. J.* 1968, **55**, 86.
8. Barnard, G. O. *J. Amer. Inst. Hom.* 1965, **58**, 205.
9. Boyd, W. E. Biochemical and biological evidence of the activity of high potencies. *Brit. Hom. J.* 1954, **44**, 6.

10. Heintz, E. Nouvelles expériences sur le mode d'action de dilutions successives. *IX^e Assises Scientifiques Homoeopathiques,* May 1970, 3–17.

11. Heintz, E. Measurement of the movement of fish and other animals in response to chemical stimuli. *Experimentia* 1958, **14**, 155. *Comptes Rend. Acad. Sci.* 1958, **246**, 1309; 1962, **255**, 2283; 1964, **258**, 3572. *Proc. 28th Congress for Homoeopathic Medicine, Vienna* 1973, p. 191.

12. Boiron, J. and Zervudacki, Mlle. Action of infinitesimal dilutions of sodium arsenate on the respiration of the coleoptiles of wheat. *Ann. Hom. Fr.* 1963, 738. *Rech. Exp. Mod. Hom.,* M. Plazy (ed.), 1967, p. 19.

13. Netien, g., Boiron, J. and Marin, A. Copper sulphate and plant growth. *Brit. Hom. J.* 1966, **55**, 186. *Ann. Hom. Fr.* 1966, 130. *Rech. Exp. Mod. Hom.,* M. Plazy (ed.), 1967, p. 73. Netien, G., Graviou and Marin. *Ann. Hom. Fr.* 1965, **248**, 253. *Rech. Exp. Mod. Hom.,* M. Plazy (ed.), 1967, pp. 68–72, 73–8.

14. Cier, A. et al. Experimental diabetes treated with infinitesimal doses of alloxan. *Brit. Hom. J.* 1967, **56**, 51.

15. Cier, A., Boiron, J., Vingert and Braise. Sur le traitement du diabète expérimental par les dilutions infinitésimales d'alloxane. *Rech. Exp. Mod. Hom.,* M. Plazy (ed.), 1967, 80–6.

16. Boiron, J. Action de Dilutions 5CH–7CH et 15CH de sulfate de cuivre sur la respiration de Salvinia Natans. *Proceedings International Congress, Vienna* 1973.

17. Aubin, M., Baronnet, S., Chazaud, J., Durantin, G., Villie, F. et Bastide, P. Action de diverses dilutions d'Arnica sur les taux de lactate deshydrogénase et de malate deshydrogénase du muscle de rats soumis à une épreuve d'effort. Communication faite aux XV^e Assises Scientifiques Homoeopathiques, à Dijon. 30 Avril 1976.

18. Boffa, M. C. Effets Biologiques du venin de Naja Nigricollis. *Proceedings of International Congress, Vienna* 1973.

19. Boffa, M. C. Modification du complément sérique par le venin de Naja Nigricollis (absorption per linguale de dose infinitésimale). *Ann. Hom. Fr.* 1976, **2**, 173.

20. Boffa, M. C. Experimentation du venin de Naja Nigricollis. *Ann. Hom. Fr.* 1976, **5**, 478.

21. Aubin, M. et Thèse de J. Bildet. Etude de l'action de différentes dilutions homoeopathiques de phosphore blanc sur l'hépatite toxique du rat. *La Documentation Homoeopathique, Les Laboratories Homoeopathiques de France,* 1975, **56**.

# SECTION II

# SYSTEMATIC APPROACH TO
# MATERIA MEDICA

In treating a patient homoeopathically we should always try to study the patient as a whole, and seek a remedy which covers as many as possible of the patient's leading symptoms. However, in our medical training we are taught to think of illnesses in relation to the systems of the body, although more than one may be involved. In this section I have selected some of the leading remedies of value in particular diseases, and set out some of the indications for them. Indeed, there are some remedies with particular affinities for certain organs, although many will appear under several systems. A fuller description of some of these appears in Section III.

Remember that diagnosis is still important, as this may help in selection of the remedy or may indicate the need for a conventional drug, a replacement therapy, or surgery.

## COMMON ACUTE REMEDIES

| | |
|---|---|
| Aconitum | Gelsemium |
| Antimonium Tartaricum | Hepar Sulphur |
| Arnica | Ipecacuanha |
| Arsenicum Album | Mercurius Solubilis |
| Belladonna | Nux Vomica |
| Bryonia | Phosphorus |
| Cantharis | Pulsatilla |
| Carbo Vegetabilis | Rhus Toxicodendron |
| Chamomilla | Sulphur |
| Colocynth | |

## POLYCREST REMEDIES OF WIDE ACTION

These remedies will have symptoms related to many different systems. They are frequently used and should be studied in detail:

| | |
|---|---|
| Arsenicum Album | Nux Vomica |
| Calcarea Carbonica | Phosphorus |
| Graphites | Pulsatilla |
| Ignatia | Sepia |
| Lachesis | Silica |
| Lycopodium | Sulphur |
| Natrum Muriaticum | Thuja |

# Chapter 9

# Accident and Injury Remedies

Most of this chapter was contributed by my colleague, Dr R. A. F. Jack, a general practitioner in rural practice with a wide experience of emergencies and accidents.

## ACCIDENTS AND FIRST AID

It is in the treatment of accidents, injuries and shock that homoeopathy excels all other therapies.

The Homoeopathic Materia Medica lists many remedies suitable for treating these conditions. For simplicity the writer has selected those medicines which he has found most useful for first aid use in general practice during the past twenty-five years. The dosages are those of his own preference, but are thought to be in accordance with current prescribing.

### Aconite
*Indications*
All cases of mental or physical shock or fright with any of the following symptoms: tremor, palpitations, hyperventilation or gasping for breath, tight feeling in the chest, feeling cold or hot, collapse, or obvious fright or distress.

*Examples*
'My grandmother has fallen down the front steps,' or 'The baby has fallen from her pram.'
'My son has just been scalded/run over/bitten by a dog.'
'She has just heard that her sister has died.'
'He has just had a near miss when a lorry ran out of control.'
and so on.

These are only some of the daily urgent messages a busy GP receives, and in any such emergency Aconite is indicated. The doctor should give it on arrival at the scene, not only to the patient but also to all others present who are emotionally involved. While it is acting it gives time for the doctor to assess the situation and plan treatment, including deciding what remedy should follow.

It works best in the highest potency (10M upwards) and should be repeated every 5 to 15 minutes, according to the emergency, as it is a very short-acting, though powerful medicine. Fortunately it acts very rapidly.

In summary, the more the shock or panic, the greater the need for Aconite, and the quicker it works.

## Arnica
### Indications
Bruises, sprains, contusions, head injuries, concussion and post-concussional headaches and myocardial infarction. Arnica is valuable for all the above conditions. It prevents and relieves muscle fatigue from over-exertion. The Swiss guides still chew Arnica leaves to prevent or to remove muscle aching and soreness.

### Dosage
Use in as high a potency as is available, e.g. 10M or higher; although, as with all homoeopathic medicines, it will work, when indicated, in any potency. Repeat every 15 minutes in acute conditions, and otherwise every 2 to 4 hours. Locally it can be applied in a cream, or as a compress, provided the skin is unbroken. For this purpose a solution is made from 2 to 3 ml of mother tincture (designated φ) in a cupful of cold water. Arnica in high potency is so effective when taken internally that local treatment is often unnecessary.

Aconite and Arnica between them probably are indicated in 80 per cent of all accidents or emergencies, and many doctors have been converted to homoeopathy following their initial experiments and successes with these two medicines.

## Calendula
### Indications
Cuts, lacerations, abrasions, gravel rash, burns, sore fissures and bed sores. Used as a mouth-wash it is an excellent haemostatic after dental extraction.

The marigold plant has an ancient reputation as a 'vulnerary' or 'wound healer'. It promotes the formation of healthy granulations.

### Dosage
Use internally in potency 12c to 200c, or apply locally in aqueous solution (10 drops of tincture in half a pint of water), oil, cream or ointment.

**Carbo Vegetabilis**
*Indications*
For collapse or faint. A valuable remedy in vasovagal attacks, or in more severe collapse, post-operatively or in cardiac cases, where the patient is cold, bluish, sweaty, with cold extremities, thin thready pulse and a desire for air at a window, or to be fanned.

*Dosage*
30c–10M potency, given frequently either in granules dry on the tongue or in water every 5–10 minutes until response, and then at longer intervals.

**Hypericum**
*Indications*
Nerve injuries – as in crushed finger tips, painful animal bites (dogs, cats and other pets, rodents, etc.), penetrating puncture wounds such as from splinters, thorns and nails. Post-operative pain. Lacerations.

St John's Wort, like marigold, is another plant quoted by Culpeper in his *Herbal*, which for centuries has been used to relieve painful injuries to soft parts richly supplied with nerve endings. In the case of a crushed finger tip, it would be indicated if the pain persisted. Arnica is given first, to stop the extravasation of blood beneath the nail.

*Dosage*
As for Calendula. Hypercal ointment, containing Hypericum and Calendula, is both soothing and healing.

**Ledum**
*Indications*
The chief remedy for puncture wounds, e.g. a nail into the sole of the foot. Also of value in bruising around the eye, where it seems to be even better than Arnica.

*Dosage*
30c–10M potency repeated 2–4 hourly as required.

**Rhus Tox.**
The poison ivy, in potency, is indicated for the effects of strains where the muscle stiffness and aching are temporarily relieved by movement, are worse at rest, and are worst after prolonged rest. The first movements to 'limber up' after a night's sleep are the most painful.

**Ruta**
Rue is ideal for treating strains of ligaments around joints, when the symptoms are 'like Rhus Tox. but more so'.

Both these follow Arnica and can be used in all potencies, repeating the dose every four hours until relief.

## Staphisagria
*Indications*
Useful in incised wounds and therefore after operation, especially in gynaecological repairs. It relieves pain and helps healing.

*Dosage*
30c–10M potency repeated 2 hourly for 6 doses.

## Symphytum – Comfrey or Knitbone
Used in lowest potencies (3x to 6x) Symphytum has the reputation of accelerating the union of fractures, and is also very useful in treating contusions of the eye.

## HEAD INJURIES

Where drowsiness persists despite medication with Arnica, give Opium 30c upwards, and if there is still no improvement consider the need for Helleborus. It is assumed that the practitioner would admit the patient to a neurosurgical unit for observation, should his condition warrant it.

For persistent post-concussional headaches, unrelieved by Arnica, use Natrum Sulph. 30c, increasing to 10M.

## INSECT AND PLANT STINGS, AND INSECT BITES

Homoeopathy certainly has more to offer than the old-fashioned treatments with blue bag, vinegar or lemon juice, and offers a satisfactory alternative to the conventional treatment with topical steroids and antihistamines.

Traditionally Ledum (Marsh tea) is given in low potency for bee and wasp stings, when the sting or bite is relieved by cold applications. The writer prefers to give Apis Mel. (potentised honey bee) to victims of bee stings, and Vespa Vulgaris (wasp) to those stung by wasps. In both cases, very high potencies (10M) should be used, repeated every five minutes until relief.

As a local application, a compress of Urtica Urens (see below) is very soothing, as is Hypercal ointment.

**Urtica Urens**
The nettle is effective used internally in potency, and externally as a compress, for nettle stings and any allergic urticarial reactions that simulate nettle stings.

## BURNS

Both Urtica and Cantharis cause and cure burning vesication of the skin, and accordingly are used in the homoeopathic treatment of burns. They are applied in the form of ointments and creams, or Urtica lotion (10 drops in one pint of boiled water).

Cantharis should also be given internally in the 30c potency every 15 minutes to 2 hours, according to the severity of the symptoms, until relief.

**Cantharis**
Spanish fly in 30c potency is effective in treating gnat bites, where painful blisters result which burn when touched, and where the affected skin rapidly necroses. Pyrethrum liquid is a useful deterrent against gnat bites, and should be diluted and applied to the exposed parts of the skin.

## HEATSTROKE

**Belladonna**
This is an excellent remedy for the effects of sun exposure, and rapidly controls the fever, headache and malaise. If the headache persists, use Glonoine.

## CHILLING

**Camphor**
An excellent prophylactic against the effects of being chilled, and as such is most useful for doctors who have to do night visits. A dose taken every five minutes until warmed will usually prevent a cold or diarrhoea from developing. If taken at the onset, Camphor will abort an attack of diarrhoea, if the patient feels very cold.

It is interesting to note that Camphor was one of Hahnemann's three specifics for the treatment of cholera.

# Chapter 10

# *Headache*

## CAUSES AND INVESTIGATION

It is important when faced with a patient complaining of headache to exclude causes which may require further investigation or neurosurgery.

**Extracranial**
Trauma.
Myalgia and cervical spondylosis.
Eye disease.
Herpes zoster.
Tic doloureux.
Cranial arteritis.
Polymyalgia rheumatica.
Migraine.

**Cranial**
Dental abscess.
Otitis and mastoiditis.
Sinusitis.
Disease of skull.

**Intracranial**
Traumatic
   Post-concussional syndrome.
   Haemorrhage – extradural, subdural.
Inflammatory
   Meningism and meningitis. Poliomyelitis. Abscess. Sinus thrombosis.
Vascular
   Subarachnoid haemorrhage.
Neoplastic
   Primary and secondary tumour.
   Pituitary tumour.

**Hypertensive**
Primary
    Essential hypertension.
Secondary
    Renal
    Vascular.
    Endocrine.

**Psychogenic**
Anxiety, hysteria.

Skull X-ray, lumbar puncture, electroencephalogram, brain scan and occasionally arteriography may be required to make a diagnosis. Teeth and sinuses should be examined and eyes tested. If hypertension is found this may need further investigation.

If there is a history of injury, even some considerable time before, we must consider using Arnica as a first prescription, before following up with further remedies. In cases of occipital blows on the head consider Natrum Sulph., which will often deal with the persistent headache.

Where the eyes seem to be the main cause of pain, we should consider such remedies as Ruta, Silica and Natrum Mur., after making any necessary adjustment to spectacles. These remedies all help in eye strain and weakness of muscle.

Sinusitis is of course a common source of head pain and one that is often difficult to cure by orthodox means. We have a wide range of remedies available here: Aconite, Belladonna, Bryonia, Spigelia, the Kali salts, Pulsatilla.

Apart from the conditions mentioned, many patients come with a history of migraine or of headache which has no identifiable cause, and may in some cases be psychogenic. I would like now to consider some remedies in more detail.

In homoeopathic prescribing for headache, the modalities are most important in distinguishing one remedy from another.

## ACUTE HEADACHE REMEDIES

**Belladonna**
Throbbing headache, worse on stooping, lying, jar and noise. Flushed dry face with enlarged pupils and often fever, sometimes accompanied by delirium.

**Bryonia**
Pain often right-sided but particularly worse on movement of head or eyes and better from pressure, occurring frequently in association with a

respiratory infection and cough which aggravates the pain; also of value in migraine.

### China Sulph.
Aching pain in the occiput extending over the head. Sweaty damp head. Better from cold applications, worse on turning the head or eyes and worse in the open air. Patient looks nauseated but wants to eat. Flatulence but cannot break wind (a China symptom).

### Gelsemium
This is of course the remedy for influenzal headache, dull, aching, occurring in damp mild weather and accompanied by the usual aching in the limbs, hot and cold sensations and chills up and down the back. Lack of thirst, even when febrile, and drowsiness add to this picture. The headache is relieved by passage of large quantities of pale urine.

### Glonoine
Bursting headache, sometimes brought on by exposure to heat of the sun, with pounding in the head, such as that found in men working with explosives.

### Iris Versicolor
Frontal headache or feeling of constriction of head, with bilious vomiting and nausea. may come on after mental strain, on relaxing. Headache worse at *rest,* better from motion. Useful in acute migraine.

### Magnesia Phosphorica
*Neuralgic* type of pain especially shooting on the right side, and a deeper occipital headache spreading over the head on the left.
Pain occurs after exposure to *cold* or nervous strain and excitement. Worse from cold air, touch, 9–11 a.m. or 4–8 p.m. Better from warmth, firm pressure.

### Sanguinaria
Recurring *periodic* headache, commencing in the morning and abating in the evening. A very useful migraine remedy for right temporal or frontal pain, with dizziness and sickness, better lying down and sleep. The menstrual periods are profuse and the patient feels worse before and after them. It is a remedy also for paroxysmal cough relieved by loud eructations of wind. Rheumatic pains in the right shoulder are also helped (Rhus Tox., Ferrum Met. also).
Sanguinaria can be given to migraine patients to use in the acute phase and it frequently cuts short the attacks or reduces their severity.

**Spigelia**
Shooting pain on the left side of the head extending to the face and arm, worse on motion, stooping.

## CHRONIC HEADACHE REMEDIES

In patients with persistent dull headache, or recurring headache, cure will often depend on accurate assessment of the patient's general and mental symptoms as well as the local features and modalities of the headache itself, in other words, seeking the totality of symptoms for that particular patient. The onset and possible precipitating causes and environmental and social conditions must be studied, and may indeed help in choosing the correct remedy. E.g. Opium following fright, Ignatia after grief, or Staphisagria where there is resentment.

Migraine treated between attacks in this more constitutional way will often become less frequent and may be cured.

### Argentum Nitricum
Headache resulting from excitement, mental overwork or travelling. It has a gradual onset and sudden cessation. There is tenseness, stiffness and soreness of the back of the neck, and a feeling as if the head is drawn back. The pain spreads over the head to the left temple and the scalp is tender to touch.

Worse at noon, using eyes, motion or exertion, even talking or stooping. Better from pressure and fresh air.

The typical Argentum Nit. patient is full of anticipatory fears, with churning and wind in the stomach, fear of heights and a strong liking for sugar and salt.

### Calcarea Carb.
Headaches caused by exposure to extremes of cold or heat, overeating or overdrinking.

It is often beating in character in the right temple, and associated with eructations, gastric upset or conjunctival congestion. The head is cold and damp to touch, and Calcarea patients sweat on the head and have cold clammy hands.

The headache is worse from light, stooping, walking and alcohol, better with eyes closed, lying down and sleeping. The typical Calcarea patient is stout, pale, sweaty and slow with fears and bad dreams.

### Cimicifuga (Actea Racemosa)
This remedy is apt to be neglected but it is a most useful one for headache. The pain is often occipital or pressing out or up as if the top of the head would fly off, and extending to the eyes. There is often

rheumatism in the muscles of the neck or neuralgia of the ciliary nerves. I think of it mainly as a female remedy with aggravation at the menstrual period, accompanied by black gloom. The patient may even think she is going insane.

Chilliness and tendency to take cold but prefers cool and open air for the local headache. Jerking and twitching of the muscles and changeableness in both physical and mental spheres (like Pulsatilla).

### Cocculus
Headache brought on by extreme exhaustion and anxiety in nursing a sick relative. Also with going in a car or boat – travel sickness with headache, dizziness and nausea. Congestion of the head, pressing or bursting with whirling and sickness.

This remedy also has slowing down of the faculties, great exhaustion, paralysis and numbness.

### Kali. Bich.
Headaches at the root of the nose and spreading, of great value in sinus trouble either with the typical sticky white or yellow catarrh or where there is pain, without discharge. The pain is worse on motion and stooping, better in the open air and eating, especially hot things. In migraine there is dimness of vision first, then a gap and then headache.

The patient dislikes the heat, and pains occur in spots; crusting of the nose and bleeding may occur. Pains of rheumatism often alternate with the catarrh. A yellowish appearance is characteristic of the remedy.

### Lachesis
Few of us would like to be without this valuable snake remedy. It is particularly helpful in menopausal patients and has a characteristic aggravation on first waking – the patient sleeps into the headache.

Pulsating hammering headache with purplish appearance of the face and puffy eyes: the blueness occurs in Lachesis generally with ecchymoses, congested purplish throat or legs.

This remedy is often left-sided and usually better from cold. The patient is generally worse from heat and tight constricting garments.

The mentals are marked with jealousy, suspicion and loquacity predominating, although slowness of speech and taciturnity can also occur.

### Lycopodium
This remedy is often applicable to the stresses, strains and rush of modern life. The headaches are often periodic and particularly occur when the patient is empty. He has the faint 'all gone' sensation one usually associates with Sulphur, and eating helps the Lycopodium headache. It is worse from heat, warmth of the bed and lying down, and

better from cold or cold air. Right-sided symptoms are common with this remedy. In spite of the relief from eating, these patients are easily filled up, distended and have much flatus. They love hot drinks and sweet food. Aggravation of symptoms at 4 p.m. or 4–8 p.m. is a useful guide.

Lycopodium is anxious and worried-looking, anticipates trouble and lacks confidence, although he is often intellectual and capable when the time comes. Dread of forgetting or making mistakes. Averse to company, especially new company and yet a dread of solitude. Fears of crowds, of the dark and of ghosts. Sensitive and emotional – he may weep when being thanked.

### Natrum Muriaticum

The Natrum headache is also hammering in type and often accompanied by visual disturbances, zig-zags or even loss of vision while reading, with watering of the eyes. It is usually worse from midday to evening and is aggravated by sun. The patient and her head are sensitive to noise, she feels the cold but is worse from much heat and is generally worse at the sea. This latter feature ties up with the strong liking or dislike of salt. Periodicity is a feature of this remedy in regard to many symptoms but equally to headache.

These patients often have greasy skins with a tendency to acne, and are usually worse at the menstrual period.

The mental symptoms are often difficult to extract because the patient is nervous and reticent by nature, but they may cover this up by an appearance of self-assurance. They tend to brood and harbour resentment, and the headache may occur as a result of emotional breakdown after grief or a disappointed love affair. They dislike sympathy, but at the same time crave attention which they consider due to them.

It is wise not to give this remedy in the acute phase of headache but rather perhaps its acute partner Bryonia, followed up by Natrum Mur.

### Nux Vomica

A most valuable remedy for the effects of over indulgence in eating, drinking or physical exertion. The hangover headache. But also useful with the Nux personality. The pains are often neuralgic in type and some gastric symptoms are common, and vertigo may accompany the headache. He is fond of tasty foods, spices and fat. Nux is essentially a chilly patient, sensitive to draughts and to all external impressions, light, noise and colours. He is above all irritable and fastidious.

### Pulsatilla

In general, Pulsatilla is worse from heat and relieved by motion. The headaches are throbbing, congestive in type, better from cold applications and slow movement, often associated with the menstrual period and relieved after it (like Lachesis). Girls with headache when about to menstruate. Sickness may accompany the headache. This remedy is valuable in periodic attacks or the old-fashioned acidosis resulting from too fat or rich food. The Pulsatilla patient likes sweet food and also pastries which upset, and is not thirsty even during fever. Symptoms of this remedy are often worse in the evening – the headache, the cough, the fever. There is frequently catarrh, usually yellow. Sinus conditions are helped, particularly where the pains are worse from heat. Changeableness of symptoms is characteristic – rheumatic pains, headaches, type of stool.

The mental symptoms are well known to you – gentle yielding disposition, easily weepy, wants attention and sympathy but is also touchy, jealous and irritable.

## Sepia

The headache of Sepia is often associated with nausea, and although occurring in pregnancy morning sickness, is usually better from sleep (unlike Lachesis). It is also improved by violent exertion. You will remember the tired, jaded, irritable housewife with backache, feelings of prolapse and must sit down. Yet take her out to a dance in the evening and she comes alive, her headache gone and her sparkle returned. Characteristically these patients are sallow and thin, feel the cold but are faint in hot, stuffy atmosphere and flush easily.

The mentals are again helpful – irritable, weepy, usually tidy but now indifferent to her house or her family.

## Silica

The headache of this remedy is often occipital extending over the head to the eyes, especially the right. The head is very sensitive to draughts and he wants it wrapped up tight and warm – the old gentleman who always wears a night cap. There is sometimes loss of half the field of vision and numbness of the arm. Bursting headache with sensitivity to noise, and aggravated by exertion physical and mental. Together with these local symptoms we have the Silica generals and mentals. Chilliness, clammy sweaty feet and hands, dread of failure, lack of confidence, lack of strength – exhausted by talking and therefore dislikes people, irritable, over-conscientious and resentful, and of course the tendency to sepsis. Silica is complementary to Pulsatilla.

## Sulphur

Periodic sick headaches, occurring at 7 day intervals, often preceded by flickering and zig-zags. Headaches often occur on Sundays, when the patient lies in late – it is better when he is busy and active. There is a feeling of dullness and congestion. The head is hot and burning with relief from cold applications, but otherwise the headache is better in a warm room, worse from light, stooping, jar and after eating. Redness of the face.

The Sulphur patient is usually untidy or dirty, selfish and full of theories. Some are stout, jovial and red-faced.


You will notice that many of these remedies for headaches are common polycrest remedies with a wide range of symptoms and application. They should be studied further in Section III and in other texts. Headache is a symptom appearing in many drug pictures.

# Chapter 11

# *Eye Remedies*

(This chapter was prepared by my colleague, Dr R. D. Calcott, ophthalmologist.)

Most eye conditions require specialist advice and surveillance, but homoeopathy can be of great value in both acute and chronic conditions.

## CATARACT

**Cineraria**

Cineraria $\phi$ 2–3 drops in an eye bath of boiled water once and later twice a day – continued indefinitely.

Calc. Iod. 6, Causticum 6 and Phos. 6 are useful remedies.

Give bd for 14 days with 14-day gap and alternate the remedies.

## CONJUNCTIVITIS

These are some of the remedies likely to be most useful:

**Apis Mel.**

If there is also a pale pink watery swelling of the lids.

**Argentum Nit.**

Use first in purulent cases – the conjunctiva can be scarlet red and oedematous.

**Arsenicum Alb.**

If a burning sensation is prominent.

**Calcarea Carb.**

Mostly in children and elderly patients – much stickiness of the lids on waking.

**Euphrasia**

Redness is diffuse with marked photophobia – discharges are acrid and can excoriate the lateral canthi. Usually accompanied by coryza and headache.

A most useful remedy in measles involving the eye and in hay fever. For relief of discomfort use 2–3 drops of mother tincture in an eye bath.

**Pulsatilla**
Discharges are profuse and bland – white to yellow pus. Better in the open air, worse in a warm room.

**Rhus Tox.**
Lids become very swollen, and hot tears spurt out on forcing lids open. Early orbital cellulitis.

## CORNEAL ULCER

**Hepar Sulph.**
Perhaps the most useful remedy – especially if hypopyon is present – pains are sharp, needle-like, in spasms worse at night. Worse in any draught.

**Mercurius Sol.**
If much vascularisation round the ulcer – also worse at night – patient may perspire.

**Conium**
Primary for dendritic ulcers – often with enlarged lymph glands.

**Graphites**
Where there are also marked cracks and exudates in the lateral canthi.

**Pulsatilla**
Of great value in chronic cases and acute cases in the young – eye often dry.

**Silica**
For chronic indolent cases with little vascularisation.

## DETACHED RETINA

**Apis Mel.**
For balloon detachment.

**Gelsemium**
For recurrences following surgery.

**Hypericum**
For pain following retinal surgery, especially if there has been an encircling procedure.

## DIABETIC RETINOPATHY

**Natrum Mur.**
Natrum Mur. is a key remedy for diabetes – so start with this. For retinal haemorrhages – use Lachesis 1 M and Hamamelis as above.

**Syzygium**
Syzygium $\phi$ 3 drops in water daily and indefinitely. Add the constitutional remedy if different from Natrum Mur.


# EPIPHORA

**Constitutional remedy**
The constitutional remedy followed by Thiosinaminum 3 tds for 2 weeks. Repeat the latter in 1 month and assess results after 3 months.

**Silica**
Silica 6 is very useful given in the waiting month, or in high potency instead of the constitutional remedy.


# EYE STRAIN

**Pilocarpus Mur.**
Despite correct glasses.


# GLAUCOMA SIMPLEX

Patients must of course always be under an ophthalmologist. The following regime is useful in maintaining normal tension.

**Gelsemium**
Gelsemium 6 tds for 14 days, after 7 days Gelsemium 30 tds one day. Repeat this 4 to 5 times a year. In between courses give the constitutional remedy in a 10M.

**Ruta**
For sudden high rises of pressure use Ruta 10M.


# INJURY

**Aconite**
*Flick on the eye.* Aconite 10M. 2 doses are usually sufficient.

**Arnica**
*Bruising of lids and orbit.* Arnica followed by Ledum 200.

**Symphytum**
*Pain of the bony orbit.*

## IRITIS

**Mercurius Sol., Mercurius Cor. and Hepar Sulph.**
*Acute*
Mercurius Sol., Mercurius Cor. and Hepar Sulph. cover a high percentage of cases.

**Constitutional remedy**
*Chronic or recurrent*
Here the carefully prescribed constitutional remedy is very important, and is then followed by the acute remedies. Most cases are women and Sepia is useful at some stage.

## MACULAR LESIONS

**Lycopodium**
Lycopodium 10M and the constitutional remedy followed in 2 weeks with Ledum 200.

## MEIBOMIAN CYST

**Thuja**
Thuja 30 for the average case (about the size of a pea).

**Staphisagria**
Staphisagria 200 where there is much oedema and redness.

**Baryta Carb.**
Baryta Carb. 10M for smaller harder cysts.

## RETINAL HAEMORRHAGE

**Lachesis**
Lachesis 1M followed by Hamamelis 6 tds 5 days.

## SCLERITIS

**Thuja**
Thuja is a very useful remedy, and often the only one required.

## SEBORRHOEIC BLEPHARITIS

This redness of the eyelids is often associated with seborrhoea of the scalp. The treatment of the lids is an exercise in finding the constitutional remedy. Where the constitutional picture of the following remedies fits the patient, some of the local signs are often as follows:

**Calcarea Carb.**
Lesions tend to be on the medial side of the lids, worse in the morning and sensitive to sunlight.

**Calcarea Phos.**
All lids involved, and mostly in teenagers.

**Graphites**
Crusting on the lids, with honey-like exudates and cracks in medial canthi.

**Lycopodium**
Often right eye only and some other lesion, e.g. chronic corneal ulcer.

**Natrum Mur.**
Very chronic cases with recurrent meibomian cysts.

**Nitric Acid**
Dark rings under the lids – often very purulent.

**Sulphur**
Burning sensation of eyelids, often accompanied by other skin lesions.


## SQUINT

**Gelsemium**
Gelsemium 6 tds for 2 weeks followed by Gelsemium 30.


## STYES

Pulsatilla 30 or Graphites 30.


## VITREOUS HAEMORRHAGE

**Ledum**
Ledum 3x tds for 14 days, repeat in 3 to 4 weeks.

# Chapter 12

# *Respiratory Remedies*

(Including those useful in infectious fevers, sore throats,
coughs and colds and early pneumonias.)

This group of illnesses forms the largest seen in general practice, and
nowadays is mainly treated with antibiotics and the occasional cough
medicine. It should be remembered that many of these are virus
diseases not affected by antibiotics, and although these drugs are still
important and life-saving they should be prescribed only with careful
thought and selection. In most situations the homoeopathic doctor will
be able to cure these illnesses with the indicated remedy. In certain
patients it may be necessary to add an antibiotic, after commencing
with the homoeopathic remedy, if the response is not adequate, if the
patient is very weak or the organism particularly virulent, or in the case
of active tuberculosis. The majority of patients, even with pneumonia,
will be cured rapidly by the correct homoeopathic remedy.

In cases of asthma it may be necessary to use a bronchodilator, an
inhaler or a short course of steroids, but this should always be secondary
to the selection of the well indicated remedy.

The ability of homoeopathic constitutional remedies to reduce the
recurrence rate of respiratory or throat infections, or the attacks of
asthma, is one of the most satisfying in homoeopathic prescribing.


## ACUTE COLDS

### Allium Cepa
Coryza with streaming eyes and nose, with acrid discharge from the
nose, and bland discharge from the eyes. There is sneezing and
headache and the patient is hot and thirsty, worse in a warm room,
better in open air.

### Arsenicum Album
Thin watery nasal discharge excoriating the upper lip, but nose stuffed
up. Sneezes from every change of weather. Chilly. Burnings relieved by
heat. Restless, anxious, fastidious.

### Arsenicum Iodatum
Corrosive, burning, pouring nasal discharge. Sneezing which aggravates. Dislike of excessive heat, restless.

### Euphrasia
In these cases the lachrymation is acrid and the nasal discharge bland. Worse from light, warmth and better in the dark. Coryza worse in the night and lying down, but cough worse by day and better lying down.

### Natrum Muriaticum
Abundant nasal discharge and lachrymation. Sneezing violent. Dry cracked lips with herpes. Severe headache worse from heat, better from cool. Again irritable, and dislikes being disturbed.

### Nux Vomica
Patient is tucked up in bed with clothes all round, even over his head. Shivers if uncovered. Aching all over, sweaty. Slight sore throat, dirty brownish tongue. Desire – warm drinks. Very irritable.

## CROUP
### Aconite (see page 69, and below)
Effects of fright or exposure to dry cold. The first stages of croup or fever. restless, fear, thirst, worse in the evening, lying on the left side, in a warm room, better from uncovering.

### Hepar Sulphuris
Starts with a cold, blocked nose, thin irritating discharge – yellow green. Sensitive to draughts, irritable, worse in cold dry weather; cough when any part of the body is exposed. Sharp sticking pains (see Throats, page 93). Desires sauces, spicy food.

### Spongia
Croupy cough, waking out of sleep with a feeling of suffocation, alarm and anxiety. Cough worse on talking, singing, swallowing or lying with the head low, lying on the right side, better from lying on the left side.

## FEVERS, COUGHS AND CHEST INFECTIONS
### Aconite
This remedy is most useful in the early stages of any fever or chill, particularly if this follows exposure to dry cold air or a frosty day. It is also indicated when a patient has had a bad fright or shock.

The onset of symptoms is sudden and is usually accompanied by fear, restlessness and anxiety; a child with a sudden fever, with a very red throat, burning dryness of the mouth and thirst for cold drinks. The symptoms are worse in the evening, in a warm room or lying on the left side, and the patient wants to throw off the bedclothes. The eyes are suffused, the pulse bounding, but the pupils not dilated. The suddenness of onset and fear are the chief characteristics, but it will often abort a cold or sore throat if given early enough.

## Antimonium Tartaricum

This if often a remedy of extreme cases of pneumonia, capillary bronchitis or left heart failure. The patient is bluish, pale, cold and sweaty but dislikes stuffiness or being wrapped up. The tongue is dry and white but without thirst (Pulsatilla, Gelsemium). There is rattling of mucus up and down the bronchial tree with a feeling of oppression or suffocation – this rattling is a leading indication for the remedy. (See also Ipecacuanha.) He may be stuporose, but want to sit up, and there is a lack of reaction.

## Belladonna

The features which suggest this remedy are those associated with overdose of atropine or the typical scarlet fever picture.

There is a high fever often accompanied by delirium, clouded sensorium, bounding pulse, with twitching and jerking, flushed dry face, circumoral pallor, dilated pupils, dry red throat and exudate with raised papillae on the tongue, and sometimes a scarlatiniform rash. In this case the patient is better from warmth and dislikes being uncovered, the opposite of Aconite. There is frequently a throbbing headache, worse from light, jar, being disturbed, and better from pressure, wrapping up the head. Belladonna may also be indicated for a headache of this type without a fever.

The patient may be in the early stages of tonsillitis or otitis media (the drum may in fact be red), or the start of an infectious fever. If the symptoms are as described this remedy will often stop the condition developing.

Local inflammatory states with red, hot, swollen, dry appearance are also helped. More toxic than Aconite.

## Bryonia

The characteristics of this remedy are stitching pains which are worse from any movement, dryness of mucous membranes and desire for large cold drinks. The aggravation from movement may apply to the pain of a pleurisy or pneumonia, to a headache or to a rheumatic or neuralgic pain. Pain in the chest is better from pressure and from lying on the affected side.

The patient is irritable, dislikes being moved or disturbed – even babies can demonstrate this symptom. The mouth and lips are dry, the tongue white, and thirst is present for large cold drinks. There is often a hard dry cough, which is painful and may cause stitching pain in the chest, or headache. The symptoms and signs are frequently more marked on the right side.

Bryonia is helpful in certain cases of measles before the rash has appeared and may encourage the rash to develop, after which the patient generally feels better.

### Carbo Vegetabilis
Characteristically the remedy for collapse or faint, with cold extremities, sweat and blue appearance, but wanting to be fanned or have the window open to get fresh air.

Also of value in capillary bronchitis, with burning in the chest, chilliness, and sometimes spasmodic cough, which makes the patient red in the face (whooping cough). Dry tongue with yellow coating and a good deal of flatulence.

### Causticum
This remedy is frequently indicated in laryngitis and tracheitis, after exposure to cold frosty weather and dry cold wind.

Hoarseness worse in the morning. (Phosphorus worse in the evening.)

Burning rawness down the trachea, with loss of voice. Inability to raise sputum, which slips back. Cough relieved by sips of cold water. Urine spurts on coughing.

These patients tend to be sallow and sickly-looking, and are often irritable, weepy, despairing and full of fears and apprehension.

### Ferrum Phos.
Early stages of inflammatory disease, especially respiratory, with fever, deep substernal soreness and painful laryngotracheal cough and epistaxis. There is alternating flush or pallor, for no apparent reason, and often an intolerance of eggs. They are more alert than Belladonna, do not have dilated pupils and have a thready weak pulse. This remedy does not have the restless anxiety of Aconite, the burning of Belladonna or the intense thirst of Phosphorus. It is indicated where the symptoms are more obviously respiratory, rather than a simple sore throat.

### Ipecacuanha
Sudden onset of respiratory infection or asthma, with rattling mucus or wheezing, *nausea* usually with a clean tongue, spasmodic cough with vomiting. Bright red blood from nose, lungs or stomach.

### Kali Carbonicum
This remedy is valuable in the acute chest infection or in the asthmatic or chronic bronchitis.

The patient is chilly and the pains are stitching, knife-like in character, worse at rest, from cold, pressure, lying on the affected side, and the surface is sensitive to pressure and touch. (Bryonia is better from rest and pressure.)

There is a characteristic 3 a.m. aggravation, the asthmatic case waking at this hour and leaning forward to obtain relief. The Kali Carb. case does not like the cold drinks of a Phosphorus patient. There is a lot of flatulence and belching of wind. There is the weakness which is present in all the Kali salts, and they are irritable, sensitive, drab uninteresting people, full of fears of the future, of death and ghosts.

## Natrum Sulphuricum
A remedy with aggravation from damp weather or warm, damp atmosphere.

The cough is loose with greenish sputum, soreness and great pain, especially in the left lower chest. There is a 4 a.m. aggravation of symptoms, although morning aggravation with depression and diarrhoea after rising are also present. These patients are depressed and may suffer from headaches, particularly following a head injury.

## Phosphorus
This remedy is invaluable in the early stages of pneumonia or bronchitis. The patient is restless, nervous, fearful of the dark or being left alone. He wants company and the reassurance of someone holding his hand. There is tightness of the chest with a hard painful cough, aggravated by cold air or laughing, sputum which is beginning to be bloodstained, and a marked thirst for large cold or iced drinks. Notice here the difference in the mental state of Bryonia and Phosphorus, the one irritable and resenting interference, the other fearful and anxious and wanting company. Although thirsty, the Phosphorus patient is often sick, bringing up the drinks a short time after swallowing them. Again the right lower lobe is often affected, and the patient cannot lie on the left side.

The physical appearance of the patient may also be a guide in selecting this remedy, either slim with brown eyes and long eyelashes, or red-haired with freckles.

## Pulsatilla
This remedy is most useful in catarrhal conditions, recurring colds, sinusitis and asthma, but it is also a good acute remedy in respiratory illness, if the symptoms indicate.

There is a characteristic absence of thirst even when the patient is fevered (see also Gelsemium, Apis).

The cough tends to be worse in the evening, dry during the night and loose in the daytime, with yellow nasal catarrh or sputum. The patient dislikes a hot atmosphere and the cough is also worse in a warm room. The eyes may be sticky and sore, sometimes with styes or blepharitis, and this is frequently seen in cases of measles, where Pulsatilla is most valuable. It will not necessarily abort the measles, but it will hasten recovery with fewer complications of ear or chest.

These patients are weepy and want attention, although they are often jealous when others receive attention in the family.

Appearance may be helpful here too, the fair haired, blue eyed, rather shy person.

# INFLUENZA

## Baptisia
Severe flu and even pneumonia, typhoid states with high fever and rapid progression to a stuporose state. There is a red or dusky complexion and the mouth is often coated and offensive (like Mercurius). Gastric symptoms are common with diarrhoea, vomiting and great prostration. Again there is a sore bruised feeling and the patient may complain of his limbs being 'scattered about'. Intense thirst and profuse sweat may also occur.

## Eupatorium Perfoliatum
The chief characteristic in this type of flu is the intense bone pains, as if they were broken. The patient hardly dares to move because of the pain (quite unlike Pyrogen). There is bursting headache worse on movement, soreness of the eyeballs and shivers and chills in the back. There may be bilious vomiting and usually marked thirst (unlike Gelsemium).

## Gelsemium
This is the most frequently used flu remedy, particularly in epidemics occurring in mild damp weather. The onset is slow with aching in the muscles and stiffness in the cervical region. There is extreme weakness, trembling of the limbs and apathy; benumbed. Shivers and chills run up and down the spine, there is a dull headache in the forehead and occiput with pain in the eyeballs and even ptosis and double vision. The tongue is dirty, but there is absence of thirst even during fever (Pulsatilla, Apis). The patient feels better in the open air and after urination – he may pass large quantities of pale urine, which relieves the headache.

## Pyrogen
Flu cases requiring this remedy are characterised by extreme restlessness and violent pulsations. The pulse may be fast with a low fever, or there may be a high temperature with a slow pulse. This dissociation is often an indication for Pyrogen. Extreme chilliness occurs with chills in the back and limbs. The patient feels bruised and beaten and the bed

feels hard, bursting headache, and above all inability to be still with the pains and restless feeling. Pyrogen is also a remedy for septic fevers and certain cases of pneumonia.

### Rhus Toxicodendron
Although often thought of for cases of rheumatism this remedy has a definite place in the treatment of influenza. The aches and pains of Rhus are characteristically worse when the limbs or body are kept still, and improve on moving them, although after a short time the patient becomes tired and stops. The restlessness then comes on again. There is stiffness on first moving or in the morning.

Damp cold weather aggravates the symptoms. There is fever, thirst, redness of the tip of the tongue and aching in the bones in flu. In the confused toxic state the patient may fear he is being poisoned.

## SORE THROATS
### Baryta Carbonica
Sore throat occurring after getting the feet wet, recurring tonsillitis with persistently enlarged glands. There is a raw scraping or shooting pain aggravated by empty swallowing. Chilliness with offensive foot sweat, salivation, hoarseness and foul taste. The patient tends to be soft, flabby and pale, there is often mucus in the nose and throat and noises in the ears, worse on chewing and better from lying down.

### Belladonna
Sudden onset of sore throat with red, inflamed appearance, strawberry tongue and the accompanying dry flush, circumoral pallor. The pupils are dilated and the fauces are dry with difficulty in swallowing. In children the fever may be accompanied by delirium and hallucinations.

### Hepar Sulphuris
These cases again have offensive discharge and profuse sweating night and day. The throat symptoms are characterised by a splinter-like pain, as if a fish bone were sticking in the throat, and sensitivity to touch. This sensitiveness applies to any septic lesion in the Hepar case. He is usually also sensitive mentally – irritable, impetuous, angry, made worse by a word, a touch, a breath of air or pain. There is a general aggravation in dry cold and amelioration in wet weather, and a liking for pickles, vinegar and often fat food.

### Lachesis
Sore throat on the left side, or beginning on the left and moving to the right, again extremely sensitive to touch and worse from a hot drink and better from cold. Congested blue appearance of the throat with dislike

of any constriction round the neck. Swallowing liquids or empty swallowing is more difficult than swallowing solids. Marked aggravation after sleep. In fever the patient may be loquacious or drowsy, with suspicion of being poisoned.

### Lycopodium
Useful in right-sided sore throats better from warm drinks. The patient is typically anxious with a worried frown.

### Mercurius Solubilis
To prescribe this remedy in sore throat, the mouth must be dirty, offensive and moist, the tongue being coated with the imprint of the teeth round the edge. Drenching sweats without relief, and worse at night and from the heat of the bed, are characteristic. Creeping chilliness is present and, although salivating, he is still thirsty. Mucopurulent discharge from the nose with rawness of the nostrils.

### Phytolacca
The throat here is dry, rough, congested and dark red. On swallowing, the pains shoot upwards to the ears like electric shocks. There may be ulceration of the throat and the pain is aggravated by hot food or drink. There is a general aggravation of all symptoms from cold, damp cold weather and at night. The neck is often stiff and there may be an irresistible inclination to bite the teeth together.

The five following *infectious fevers* may usefully be considered here.

# CHICKENPOX
### Antimonium Tartaricum
Where spots are slow to come out, and especially if bronchitis is present (see pages 89 and 116).

### Rhus Toxicodendron
Vesicular eruptions with marked itching.

# MEASLES

Consider Pulsatilla, Euphrasia, Sulphur.
Bryonia if you suspect he is incubating it, is fevered and coughing, but the rash has not yet appeared.
Morbillinum (the nosode) after the acute phase is past.

## MUMPS

Mercurius with salivation, offensive sweat.
Pilocarpine: almost a specific remedy in mumps.
Pulsatilla with orchitis present.


## WHOOPING COUGH
**Carbo Vegetabilis**
Already mentioned (see page 90).

**Drosera**
Is the most commonly indicated remedy, with spasmodic cough and
  vomiting worse after midnight.
This remedy is also of value in tuberculous conditions.

**Cuprum Metallicum**
Where spasms are extreme and may lead to convulsions.

**Pertussin** (the nosode)
To be used either as a prophylactic for other members of the household,
or as a follow-up remedy after the acute phase, where cough persists.


## GLANDULAR FEVER

There is no specific homoeopathic remedy for this condition, but
patients present with fever, rash, small glands in the neck, and often a
very painful throat with inflammation and exudate. Remedies to consider are Belladonna in the early stage, and Mercurius Cyanatus or
Solubilis if the mouth is dirty with salivation, bad breath and sweating.
Calc. Phos. can be helpful to follow, for the glands, and a dose of
Glandular Fever Nosode 30 will often help the rather slow con-
valescence.


## TEETHING
**Chamomilla**
This is a remedy no doctor should be without in acute illness, especially
in children. The child is irritable, wanting to be carried about, or
bounced up and down. Whenever he is put down he starts to roar again.
Teething, one cheek bright red. Dry cough in sleep. Burning hot feet.
Stools often green and offensive, with colic.

# Chapter 13

# *Cardiovascular Remedies*

Many homoeopathic doctors use some of the conventional cardiac drugs in certain situations, but whenever possible these should always be supplementary to a homoeopathic remedy.

In cardiac failure, drugs such as digoxin or diuretics may be needed. We are all aware now of the need to restrict the dosage of digitalis, especially in the elderly, because of toxic effects, and there are some patients who genuinely cannot tolerate any of the cardiac glycosides. Remedies such as Apis, Crataegus and Convallaria may have sufficient diuretic effect, but may need to be supplemented by frusemide, bendrofluazide or aldactone.

In hypertension there is still considerable debate about the importance of lowering the blood pressure level, particularly in elderly patients. Here again a diuretic or beta-blocking drug should only be used if adequate response is not obtained by remedies like Crataegus, or by constitutional prescribing.

In angina and myocardial ischaemia there are a number of effective homoeopathic remedies, although, in an acute infarction, intensive care and resuscitation procedure may be life-saving. Aconite, Carbo Veg. and Arsenicum Album can have dramatic effects in acute situations.

In more chronic states, again, look at the patient as a whole. Take into account his general symptoms, his emotional and mental symptoms as well as his pain, breathlessness or oedema, and try to select a remedy covering as wide a range of symptoms as possible.

## TINCTURES

**Adonis Vernalis**
After rheumatism or influenza. Low vitality, weak heart, slow weak
pulse. Cardiac asthma. Irregular heart – possible substitute for
digitalis.

**Convallaria Majalis** (Lily of the Valley)
Dilatation of the ventricles – oedema. 'Tobacco' heart 'as though heart
stopping and starting'.

**Crataegus Oxycantha** (5 drops tds in water.)
For weak or irregular heart. Arteriosclerosis and chronic cardiac states. Myocarditis, worse in a warm room, better in the fresh air.

**Iberis** (Tincture of 1x potency.)
Palpitation from slightest exertion, laughing or coughing – darting pains in heart. Worse on lying down, on left side, exertion, warm room.

## ANGINA

**Cactus**
Constriction, squeezing of heart. Iron band prevents heart moving. Violent irregular beats, worse lying, especially on left side. Hot, sweaty. Fear and distress worse at 11 a.m. or p.m.

**Kalmia**
Violent palpitations with faint feelings, or slow feeble pulse.
Wandering rheumatic pains in the heart and left arm.
Heart disease resulting from rheumatic fever, especially where rheumatic symptoms are better and heart symptoms are worse (the wrong direction for cure).
Symptoms worse if leaning forward.

**Lachesis** (Surukuku or bushmaster snake)
Useful in angina or cardiac failure if symptoms match.
The main characteristics of this remedy are blueness of appearance or local lesions, aggravation of symptoms after sleep, tendency to left-sided symptoms, aggravation from heat, and palpitation and symptoms of choking, out of proportion to the local signs.
Choking feeling is aggravated by touch, hot drinks, empty swallowing.
These patients are often loquacious, jealous and suspicious.

**Latrodectus Mactans**
Violent precordial pains extending to the left arm and fingers, with numbness – radiating to the abdomen. *Cramping* in quality.
Quick, thready pulse.
Anxiety, cold sweat, gasping respiration.
May yell with pain.

**Lilium Tigrinum**
Dull gripping pain in chest and right arm, worse from consolation, warmth, lying down and pressure. As if heart grasped violently and then slowly released – wakes her.

Violent palpitation.

Weepy, *hurried,* bearing down like Sepia.


**Lycopus** (In potency or tincture.)

Paroxysmal tachycardia. *Protruding* eyes, *goitre.* Tumultuous sensation in cardiac region.

Pale, restless. Throbbing worse lying on the *right* side.


**Naja** (Cobra)

Tremblings worse from sleep, tight things (Lachesis).

Choking, grasping sensation of the throat – irritating dry cough.

Oedema, but *not* haemorrhage or purpura. Surging of blood upwards.

*Nerve* lesions, even bulbar palsy – paralysis of speech, swallowing with marked salivation.

Broods over imaginary problems, suicidal depression, dreads to be left alone.

Pain in the left temple and left orbital region extending to the occiput with nausea and vomiting.

Violence of heart beat – audible; valvular lesions, cannot lie on the left side. Weight on the heart. Stitching pain with *numbness* of left arm and hand.

Angina extending to the nape of the neck and left arm with anxiety and fear.

Cold body but head hot; worse in warm room; slow weak irregular pulse.

Endocarditis and myocarditis. Dull aching pain in back in cardiac cases.

Also hay fever, raw larynx and trachea and even asthma, especially cardiac.


**Oxalic Acid**

Severe pain, sharp lancinating, extending through to the back on the left side. Worse on movement.

Mottled appearance. Dyspnoea – sharp pain on breathing.


**Spigelia**

Violent beating of the heart so that he can hear the pulsation – see the beats.

Palpitation, worse on sitting down and leaning forwards.

Must lie on the right side with head very high.

Stitching pains, worse from motion. Pericarditis.

Left orbital stabbing pain.

**Spongia**
Oppression with cardiac pain worse if lying with head *low.*
Constriction, palpitation – sudden waking with suffocation, alarm and
anxiety – sweaty. Sensation as if heart is swelling and would burst.
Barking cough.

## HEART FAILURE

**Ammonium Carbonicum**
Pale, worse in cold wet weather, better in dry weather.
Want of energy, power, strength and tone.
Played out – mind and body (after serious illness or flu).
Uneasiness, anxiety, weakness.
Often women; nervous, venous and lymphatic constitution, fat, flabby.
Oppressive fullness in forehead, worse from cold. Nosebleeds on waking
in morning.
Stuffed coryza at night.
Emphysema and bronchitis – mucus and rattling like Antimonium Tart.
Asthma worse in a *warm* room, 3 a.m.
*Heart* dilated – breathless and palpitation on exertion, worse in a hot
room.
Faintness with hysteria (nasal effect of Ammonia).
Also audible pulsation with great prostration.
*Stomach* fullness worse while or after eating.
Acrid fluids – nose, saliva, stool, leucorrhoea.
As an antidote to Lachesis – should not be used after it.

**Antimonium Tartaricum**
This remedy mentioned under respiratory remedies is the remedy to
think of in acute left heart failure. Accumulation of mucus in the
bronchial passages with rattling respiration, and inability to
expectorate. Worse from heat.
Patient is pale, or cyanosed, cold, drowsy and has intense nausea with
prostration.

**Apis** (Obtained from the bee sting poison.)
Of value in oedema and heart failure.
Affects skin, mucous membranes, but also meninges, pericardium.
Swelling, stinging, burning, redness, oedema, urticaria. Worse from
*heat,* after sleep. Better from cold air, cold applications.
Sudden onset. Puffy eyelids.
*Thirstless* even in oedema or fever.
*Throat* oedematous, worse from heat – may be painless or stinging,
burning.

*Mind* Sad, tearful, depressed, constant weeping, no sleep from worry-
  ing. Irritable, suspicious and jealous. Joyless, indifference.
Fear of death. Restless and anxious.

## Arnica
Although thought of as an injury remedy, it has a much wider action.
  Used for the effects of 'injury' after myocardial infarction or cere-
  brovascular accident.
The patient and his heart are weak and tired.
Aching as if bruised – bed feels too hard.
May say he is fine when he is in fact seriously ill.

## Arsenicum Album
For acute cardiac situations with symptoms occurring at midnight or
  1 a.m. Sensation of weight, pressure or constriction of the chest.
Anxious, fearful, restless, prostration, with burning pains, thirst for
  warm drinks, vomiting and diarrhoea.
Very chilly, but wants head cool.

## Carbo Vegetabilis
The homoeopathic 'corpse reviver', a remedy widely used in situations
  of collapse, faint vasovagal attacks, coronary attacks, cardiac failure.
The patient is collapsed, cold, sweaty and pale, with thin, thready pulse,
  but gasping and wanting the window opened.
Nose and lower legs particularly cold.
Sluggishness, distended veins with burning sensations, although cold.
  Distension and flatulence.

## Kali Carbonicum
Has the weakness associated with all potassium salts.
The heart is weak with irregular, intermittent pulse. Always chilly.
Characteristic stitching pains, especially in the chest in heart or lung
  affections.
Shortness of breath, must sit up, worse at 3 a.m.
Puffiness of the upper eyelids.
Irritable, very sensitive to noise, and full of fears.

## Laurocerasus (Distillation of common laurel leaves.)
Contains hydrocyanic acid.
Coldness – want of heat, want of reaction, *not* helped by warmth.
Feeble circulation and weak heart, which may be slow or irregular.
Cyanosis of the newborn and in cardiac cases. Cold, clammy feet and
  legs.
In *warm* room patient breaks out in cold sweat and *feels nausea*.
Prolonged fainting. Spells of profound sleep.

*Gasping* for breath. Any effort aggravates the chest pain. Cheyne Stokes dyspnoea.

Twitching of face or limbs.

Suffocating feeling – *better* from lying down (Psorinum).

Vertigo – must lie down.

Aching pains in frontal bone (as if brain fell forward).

*Dryness* of tongue.

Drinks roll audibly down to intestines. Pains in lower abdomen, with loose green stools.

Irritating cough of heart cases worse on lying, but constriction of larynx is better from lying.

Paralysis of bladder with either retention or feeble stream and dribbling.

# Chapter 14

# *Gastrointestinal Remedies*

In approaching the treatment of this group of diseases, the physician must use his clinical acumen, accurate history-taking and, if indicated, investigations such as barium meal or enema, sigmoidoscopy, and endoscopy, to try to establish a diagnosis. Although this may not alter his therapeutic approach in dyspepsia, peptic ulcer, colitis or diverticular disease, it will help to eliminate the possiblity of neoplasm or gross ulceration where surgery may be required.

If a patient presents with a perforation, severe haemorrhage, obstruction or acute appendicitis, a surgical opinion should always be sought. Prescribing of homoeopathic injury remedies before and after operation can greatly ease the patient's discomfort and speed recovery, e.g. Arnica, Staphisagria, Carbo Veg. and Calendula.

Diet plays an important role in gastric and bowel disorders and the use of bran and high roughage diets is of value in diverticular disease and certain kinds of colitis. A gluten-free diet in coeliac disease, or avoidance of certain sugars, where there is intolerance, is essential, but remedies will often enable patients to absorb or utilise foods more efficiently.

Treatment of peptic ulcer still presents great problems, although drugs like cimetidine and the liquorice preparations have improved healing. Relapses still occur on discontinuing treatment, and a homoeopathic remedy, by improving the patient's health as a whole, is more likely to effect a cure. Some patients may require surgery.

In gallbladder disease, inflammation responds well to our remedies, but if stones are present with recurring acute attacks of pain and sickness, operation may be needed. Many patients who are a poor operative risk or who are elderly may live quite comfortably with their stones under homoeopathic care.

In acute situations parenteral fluids, blood or intravenous feeding should be given on the usual medical indications.

Early diagnosis of neoplasm with surgical removal still offers the best hope of cure, but homoeopathy can greatly improve the patient's health and often keep him comfortable with a minimum of sedation, even in advanced disease.

This section includes remedies often of value in dyspepsia, peptic ulcer, colitis, diverticulitis, diarrhoea and piles.

While these remedies have local symptoms related to stomach and bowel, try to look at the patient as a whole in his general symptoms and mental symptoms. This may help you to select the correct remedy.

Tyler's *Pointers to the Common Remedies, Number 2* is a valuable reference book for these conditions. Symptoms related to stomach and bowel will also be found in the pictures of remedies in Section III.

## STOMACH REMEDIES

**Anacardium orientale** (Juice of the Marking Nut)
This remedy is often of value in gastric complaints where the pain occurs when the stomach is empty. There is relief from eating for 2 or 3 hours, and then pain recurs. (In Nux Vomica the discomfort is worse while digestion is occurring for several hours after eating.)

There is a sensation of a *plug* in the anus, with urge to stool but not sufficient power to carry it out.

Sensation of a hoop or *band* round the affected part.

The other main sphere of action of this remedy is the *mental one*.

Impaired memory; sensation as if he is double – one part seeking to do good and the other evil. A lowering of moral control with irresistible desire to curse, swear or do violence to loved ones; feelings of unreality (Medorrhinum), marked irritability, irresolution or cannot decide. Full of fears that he is pursued, that something will happen.

Like Rhus Tox. in skin eruptions – itching, vesicular eruptions.

**Arsenicum Album**
This is a frequently used remedy in acute gastroenteritis with both vomiting and diarrhoea. There is dryness of the tongue with thirst for small drinks, preferably warm. The stools are offensive, frequent, watery, *excoriating* and *burning*, and better from heat. There is prostration after stool, and profuse sweat.

The gastric upset usually follows a chill, cold drinks, fruit, spoiled food, teething or food poisoning. The Arsenicum mental symptoms must be present – prostration, fear and restlessness. This remedy will also work best in an Arsenicum type – extremely tidy, anxious, restless people.

**Argentum Nitricum**
Overworked, overtired persons with headache, mental exhaustion, marked anticipatory upset leading to diarrhoea, and a constant hurried feeling.

Flatulent dyspepsia and gastric ulcer with considerable wind and distension. Stools are greenish, like chopped spinach.

Dislike of hot atmosphere, stuffy places, crowds and high places. Pains in abdomen immediately after eating, relieved by vomiting. During the acute phase there is a desire for cold or iced food and drink. Strong liking for sweet food, especially sugar and also salt or strong-tasting foods, but sweet may upset.

The tongue is smooth and red during chronic diarrhoea but often pale, flabby and dry with gastric upsets.

## Carbo Vegetabilis

This is one of the great flatulent remedies (see also China, Lycopodium, Argentum Nit.). The patient feels blown up and distended and is relieved by eructation or passage of flatus. Again, rich food or cold drinks on a hot day upset.

The patient is usually icy cold, sweaty, with coldness of the extremities and nose. He may be faint and looks pale or blue in colour.

There are small, watery, excoriating stools with burning in the rectum and odourless flatus.

## Graphites

This remedy is particularly applicable in persons who are pale, overweight, despondent and lacking in energy. They are hesitant and find decisions difficult to make. Unusual stress upsets them.

Chilly patients, but with dislike of stuffy atmospheres. The stomach symptoms are heartburn, eructation, sick feelings, griping pains with faintness and sometimes vomiting of blood. The pains occur about 2 hours after meals and are relieved by eating, by warm drinks, by milk and by lying down. There is a dislike of sweet foods. Constipation without any urge and then large pale stool with mucus and colic.

Graphites cases very often have a skin lesion or a history of past skin eruptions, or fissure and piles.

## Lycopodium

This remedy is useful in dyspepsia and in peptic ulcer. There is much heartburn with eructations and pain in the right hypochondrium (duodenal or gallbladder conditions especially). The symptoms tend to be worse in the late afternoon, 4–8 p.m., and distension of the abdomen is a predominant symptom, with desire to loosen the clothes. Patients may feel hungry but are easily filled up after a small quantity of food. There is often considerable wind in the bowel with flatus, and constipation of a spasmodic kind with pain.

There is a strong liking for sweet food and for hot drinks, but the headache or skin lesions in these cases are usually better from cold and worse from heat.

This is often the remedy for the intellectual type of patient with a tendency to worry over little things, to lack confidence, although in fact they are perfectly capable when the time comes. There is fear of the dark, of crowds, and of being completely alone, although they like to be on their own, provided there is someone in the next room. Symptoms and signs are very often right sided in Lycopodium cases.

## Natrum Carbonicum

These patients often resemble a Sepia case, pale, sallow, thin, stooped and timid. There is inability to concentrate, depression and dislike of mental effort, and lack of interest in the family. Symptoms often occur as a result of overwork. They are sensitive to noise, light, and tastes, although the sense of smell is poor, due possibly to catarrh which is frequent and yellow in colour. Chilly but worse in extreme heat, exposure to hot sun or electric thunderstorms.

There is a marked intolerance of milk and aggravation from starchy foods, vegetable and fat, causing flatulence and dyspepsia with acid mouthfuls. They like sweet foods and are often greedy and constantly nibbling. Eating helps for a short time – hunger at 5 a.m. or 11 p.m. (night hunger in pregnancy).

Constipation present or greyish diarrhoea when gastric upset: jaundice.

Herpes of the lips and hair margin, and dry skin with cracks at the finger tips.

## Nux Vomica

This is one of the most frequently used remedies for gastric upset, particularly when it follows indiscretion of eating or drinking or the effects of stress or overwork. The patient wakes up with a headache and a bad taste in the morning.

There is much retching with peristaltic movements and distension, usually 2–3 hours after food – vomiting tends to relieve the symptoms.

Desire for rich and tasty foods, pickles etc., which upset as the patient is usually 'livery'. There may be flushing or fainting while eating.

Constipation is common with incomplete motions and much straining. It is also useful in colicky diarrhoea, with hard lumps with watery motions and mucus such as is found in colitis.

The general and mental symptoms are a useful guide to Nux Vomica. Chilliness, with aggravation from draughts, but a dislike of hot stuffy atmosphere. Sensitivity to smells, noise and pain, and above all irritability and fastidiousness (one of the extremely tidy remedies like Arsenicum Album).

## Phosphorus

This remedy is useful in vomiting, and in haematemesis where there is marked thirst for cold or iced drinks. These are gulped down, and after a short time vomited up again. Burning in stomach, weak empty sensation in the abdomen. Pains better for cold food, ice cream.

Diarrhoea – profuse stool, blood in stools, sphincter relaxed with involuntary stool.

The Phosphorus patient is tall, thin, artistic, with fine dark hair (sometimes red hair), sensitive and full of fears. Note burnings better from cold (Arsenicum better from warm).

## Pulsatilla

The Pulsatilla patient is usually gentle, mild and yielding, with tendency to weep and need for affection, although they can be very jealous. They are often plump and fair-haired. Changeableness is a marked symptom. The gastric symptoms are as follows.

Dryness of the mouth with absence of thirst, and persistent taste of food hours after eating. Pains, sickness and diarrhoea occur from taking very cold or iced food or fruit, especially when overheated, but the heartburn and rawness are aggravated by warm food. These patients often like rich food, pastries and sweet things, but they are upset by them. There is a livery tendency, and Pulsatilla is valuable in the cyclical vomiting or acidosis of children which is usually aggravated by cream, chocolate or rich food.

The stools are variable, constantly changing. There may either be burning diarrhoea with mucus, worse at night, or constipation with ineffectual urging as in Nux Vomica.

There is a general aggravation from hot atmosphere.


## BOWEL REMEDIES

### Aloes

Like Sulphur, worse from heat, venous congestion.
Large piles, blue, painful, better from cold applications.
Rumbling in abdomen, colic and urge to stool.
Distension, fullness, liver congestion. Eating causes stool.
Yellowish, thin burning stools, with mucus, driving him out of bed.
    Lack of control.
Headaches worse from heat.

### Chamomilla

This is the remedy most commonly associated with teething in children, with irritability and desire to be carried about. It is also useful in diarrhoea with teething. One cheek flushed. Thirst with a coated tongue. Sour vomiting and hot sweat at night. Sensitive to pain.

The stools are green, small, frequent, offensive or like rotten eggs with mucus. There is redness and puffiness around the anus.

## China

This is one of the windy remedies, with distension not relieved by flatulence or passage of flatus. The patient is often pale, cold and weak, but does not want air (opposite of Carbo Veg.). A remedy indicated after loss of fluid (diarrhoea, bleeding, vomiting).

Diarrhoea tends to be worse in the early morning or after midnight, watery, undigested with mucus and flatus. The stool may be either painless or irritating, but not usually burning.

Colic is better from warmth and lying and worse on eating, especially fruit. There is thirst for sour drinks.

## Colocynth

Violent griping, twisting *colic* pains in central abdomen; frequent passage of flatus with relief.
Stitching pains in the sides. Abdomen greatly distended and painful.
The colic makes him double up and is only relieved by pressing on the bowels and doubling up. Paroxysms of colic. Frequent urging to stool.
Symptoms are often related to previous frustration or anger.

## Magnesia Phos.

Spasms of *cramp* in the stomach, griping with belching of wind, which does not relieve. (Colocynth relieved by flatus.)
Flatulent colic, forcing patient to bend double, *better* from *warmth* and rubbing.
Magnesia Phos. is worse from cold air, cold water, touch, better from heat, warmth, pressure, bending double.

## Mercurius Cor.

Diarrhoea with slimy, bloody stools, with colic and faintness and marked tenesmus during and after stool, accompanied by creeping chilliness. The other features of Mercurius may be present. Foulness and offensiveness, sweating, thirst and aggravation at night and from the heat of the bed.

## Phosphoric acid

This is a good remedy for summer diarrhoea, again from overeating, fruit or spoiled food.

The patient is pale, easily exhausted and does not want to talk. Marked apathy and indifference. There is thirst and a desire for sour things, and polyuria.

The stools are watery, *painless*, odourless and profuse, sometimes green and accompanied by flatus, and there may be rectal prolapse (note the difference from Arsenicum Album). Debilitating and exhausting.

**Podophyllum**
This is often the diarrhoea of hot weather. The patient appears ill, pale and collapsed and dark under the eyes. There is cold or hot sweat, a coated tongue and bilious vomiting. Cramps occur in the lower limbs and the colic is better from heat and pressure, and worse lying on the back.

The stools are offensive, painless with flatus and spluttering and may be yellow in colour. Diarrhoea tends to be worse at night or 3–5 a.m., and after food. Prolapse or piles may be present.

**Psorinum**
Dirty looking, rough-skinned, offensive smelling patient, sweating profusely at night.
Sleepless and hungry during the *night*. Lies on the back with arms
 abducted.
Sensitive to cold air.
Stools are liquid, very dark, horribly *offensive*, with a penetrating odour
 (of rotten eggs). Sudden and frequent evacuations, but no marked
 pain.

**Veratrum Album**
Pale, sunken face.
Excessive coldness, cold sweat of the forehead, icy sensation on the
 vertex.
Extreme thirst for cold or ice.
Copious vomiting and purging with sweat and collapse, and intense
 nausea.
Paralytic weakness and loss of power.
Violence of reactions to pain, and mania.
Diarrhoea is profuse with perspiration and icy coldness.

# PILES

**Aesculus**
This has a feeling of small sticks in the rectum, with dry, hard stools, and pains in the sacral region.

**Aloes**
See page 106.

**Collinsonia**
Where there is much bleeding, and obstinate constipation.

**Muriatic Acid**
This is for sensitive piles better from warmth, with poor muscle control of anus, prolapse and great weakness.

**Nitric Acid**
This is more indicated in fissure with knife-like pain shooting up the rectum and remaining long after stool.

**Nux Vomica**
This is a common pile remedy with much tenesmus and following indiscretions of eating. Very irritable (see page 105).

**Paeonia**
This remedy is where the piles are congested and acutely painful.

**Sulphur**
This is frequently indicated with repeated piles, local congestion and other Sulphur indications.

# Chapter 15

# *Genito-urinary Remedies*

There are a number of useful homoeopathic remedies for cystitis, retention, incontinence, renal calculi and leucorrhoea. It is important in cystitis or pyelitis to culture the urine. If your remedy does not clear up the infection quickly, especially in younger patients, further investigation or an antibiotic may be required to avoid chronic renal damage. If haematuria is present, pyelography or cystoscopy should be considered to exclude a neoplasm. Stones may require surgical removal, but sometimes smaller ones will pass with the help of a homoeopathic remedy. In elderly men, remedies may help benign prostate enlargement for many years, without operation, but careful clinical examination and investigation is essential to exclude malignancy.

The remedies described here have useful bladder symptoms. Always remember the more general, constitutional symptoms too, as these may help in selection of the correct remedy.

## URINARY REMEDIES
### Berberis
A great remedy in renal or gallbladder colic – may help patient to pass a small renal calculus.

Soreness in renal area worse from pressure, jar of walking or in a car, but restless, because the pains are stitching and *radiate* across the back or down the ureter.

Urging and burning in bladder and urethra.

Of value in pale, gouty or rheumatic patients. Pains move about stitching and stabbing – in joints, in neck, in back, worse on stooping.

Restlessness. Pains and coldness in head. Characteristically radiating pains from one point.

### Cantharis
Violent burning, cutting pains in bladder and urethra which get steadily worse. The patient wants something done quickly, may scream, become irritable and even insolent, and delirious in fever. These symptoms are worse in the afternoon, and the pains occur before,

during and after micturition. They are accompanied by tenesmus and only a few drops of urine pass.

Restless and very thirsty; disgust for food.

Also of value in bowel inflammation with blood and mucus, burning and distension and tenesmus (like Mercurius Cor.).

A remedy for erysipelas – red, burning and blistering – also given by mouth following burns and scalds, with intense pain and blisters. (Urtica lotion locally.)

### Causticum

A most valuable cystitis remedy, with acute sensitivity to cold. Great urgency with inability to pass urine, then later, while sitting, involuntary urination without warning. Shooting pains in the rectum when cannot pass urine.

Incontinence on coughing or exertion.

Retention of urine after operations, especially gynaecological – this remedy will often save unnecessary catheterisation.

Aggravation in cold dry winds and frost causing paralysis, especially of face, raw cough and loss of voice, and rheumatic pains.

Melancholy, anxious, irritable, full of forebodings.

### Clematis

Burning sensation at the beginning of urination – this sensation continues in the urethra for a long time after passing urine. Feels as if urethra will close up – a feeling of constriction, and the flow is very slow.

The bladder is seldom quite empty.

Small itchy crusts on the scalp, pustular rash round the loins.

Toothache, unbearable at night – want to draw in cold air or drink cold water.

Dread of being alone and yet dislikes company. Apprehension, weeping and homesick. Irritable and angry.

### Sabal Serrulata

Mainly a remedy of value in prostatic enlargement – can be given in 6x potency twice daily over long periods, sometimes enabling older men to do without operation.

These patients also get confused, depressed and irritable, want to be left to die, and get angry at sympathy.

Fear of going to sleep, because of unknown danger.

Bladder feels full – scalding urine and feeling of blockage in the meatus. Feeling as if testicles are tightly drawn up. Also pains in the head, aching in temples, especially right, with vertigo. Pains at root of nose extending up into head, or at base of skull extending down to cervical region.

**Sarsaparilla**

Pains at the *end* of micturition – urgency but little passes. Urine flows more easily on standing than sitting. White, turbid appearance of urine, with mucus.

Passes gravel or stones.

Also weakness, sluggishness, failure to heal.

Applications of heat improve but internal heat aggravates (e.g. hot food).

Like Secale, but Secale is better from local cold and uncovering.

Symptoms generally worse from walking, motion, going up and down stairs.

**Terebinth**

*Four cardinal symptoms of this remedy:*

Burnings.

Drowsiness, even when having pain.

Smooth, red, glazed tongue.

Tinkling sensation in the ears – own voice sounds unnatural and direction of sounds is disturbed.

Violent burning and cutting pains in the bladder, with smoky, bloody urine.

Similar pains in abdomen extending from left to right with distension.

Pains in kidneys worse from sitting, better from moving about.

Haemorrhages – ecchymoses, stomach and bowel, kidney and bladder.

## GYNAECOLOGICAL REMEDIES

The symptom of leucorrhoea appears in many remedy pictures. The correct remedy must cover not only the modalities of the discharge, but also some of the patient's general symptoms.

**Hydrastis**

This remedy is best known for its catarrhal symptoms, involving respiratory, gastrointestinal, urinary and genital systems.

The discharges are characteristically *ropy* and viscid.

*Leucorrhoea* is thick, yellow, and viscid, with soreness and excoriation, and vulvar itch.

The other marked symptom of Hydrastis is an empty faint feeling in the stomach with loathing of food, and obstinate constipation with no desire for stool.

## Kreosotum

*Putrid*, excoriating discharges – yellow staining, with violent itching and *burning* pain.

Offensiveness of all discharges.

Also in tooth decay with pain and bad odour.

Bleeding easily from small wounds. Profuse menses with flow heavy on lying down.

## Lilium Tigrinum

A hot type of Sepia. Usually fat and fair.

Hot and *hurried*.

Angry and bad tempered, depressed and silent, and again indifferent to her family. Feel only they can do a particular thing – no one else can.

Exacting – things revolve round her. Fear of going crazy, of what happens after death. Menses irregular, clotting, heavy. Uncontrollable sexual excitement worse before menses.

Sensation as if the whole of the inside would fall out (like Sepia).

## Mercurius

Greenish, biting leucorrhoea, with burning and desire to scratch.

Burning and urging to urinate.

Diarrhoea with urging and tenesmus, mucus and blood.

Worse from the *heat* of bed, worse at *night*.

Sweating without relief; dirty moist tongue with thirst and salivation.

## Nitric Acid

Itching, burning discharge with splinter-like pains and ulceration.

Offensive, yellowish, bloody.

The severe pains of anal fissure or piles. These patients are *chilly*, depressed, irritable, indifferent, intolerant of sympathy, and sensitive to pain, noise, touch or jar.

Profuse sweat of hands and feet.

Desire for *fat* and *salt*.

Warts.

## Pulsatilla

One of the polycrest remedies described fully in Section III, but often a female remedy.

Plump, tearful, mild, yielding person who wants sympathy, and yet is jealous and irritable too.

Chilly and yet hates warm stuffy atmosphere. Better in open air, better from slow movement. Changeable. Most discharges in Pulsatilla are bland but leucorrhoea can be excoriating, thick yellow or green. Menses are often late or absent – may help to start the period in adolescent girls.

Marked sexual excitement in male or female, and yet fear of the opposite sex.

**Sepia**
This is one of the most commonly used female remedies, with a wide variety of symptoms.

The most characteristic pelvic symptom is the 'bearing down' sensation as if the organs would prolapse – it will help to improve pelvic muscle tone in certain degrees of prolapse, but severe cases will also require operation. Low backache.

Great dryness of vagina and vulva causing discomfort on walking.

Leucorrhoea gelatinous, yellow or white, burning and excoriating.

A remedy of both heavy irregular menses, or late and absent ones.

Sudden hot flushes with weakness and faint feelings at the menopause.

The classical Sepia person is chilly, sallow, dull, irritable and indifferent to loved ones, but always better from sleep and from exercise, especially dancing, which brings her alive.

## MENOPAUSE

In the *menopause*, with flushings and emotional symptoms, we should consider remedies like:

Sepia
Lilium Tigrinum
Sulphur
Lachesis, Cenchris and Squid (Dr Blackie)
Natrum Mur.
Staphisagria

These are described in more detail in Section III.

# Chapter 16

# *Skin Remedies*

The main types of skin disease seen in general practice include the following:

1  Infective: either parasitic – scabies and pediculosis – or septic – boils and abscesses; also shingles.
2  Allergic: in this group we may include familial tendencies manifesting in atopic eczema. Allergy to local irritants, e.g. nickel, detergents, petroleum, washing and bleaching powders; industrial, such as wood shavings, sugar or flour.
3  Dermatitis due to stress.
4  Acne vulgaris and acne rosacea.
5  Psoriasis and other skin eruptions of unknown aetiology.
6  Warts.
7  Other rarer forms of skin disease.

Homoeopathic doctors are frequently faced with many of these conditions, very often after the patient has had various types of local applications, and has ceased to respond or become allergic to the treatment. Parasitic infections may require local conventional applications.

Occupational hazards, nickel, buckles, and the notorious 'whiter than white' washing powders must be eliminated. Certain foods such as peas, beans, lentils, milk, eggs, wheat flour and shellfish may be causal in eczema. It is often helpful to start a patient on a few days of water only, and then gradually to introduce vegetable and fruit juices, salads, protein and then the possible allergic foods one at a time. This will provoke an aggravation if the patient is sensitive to particular foods.

There are certain local skin appearances which may guide us to a remedy, but general and mental symptoms are often essential for cure. In the course of this case taking we may also come upon a psychological reason for the skin lesion.

Local signs of value are:

the vesicular eruptions of Rhus Tox.
the cracks and hacks of Petroleum.
the dry cracking with sticky oozing of Graphites.
the redness and intense itch of Sulphur.
the dirty, smelly lesions of Psorinum.

In homoeopathic prescribing, most physicians regard skin diseases as merely external manifestations of a deeper underlying disorder. This applies particularly to eczema, dermatitis and psoriasis. For this reason the homoeopathic doctor prefers to treat the patient with an internal remedy, based not only on the skin appearances and local symptoms, but also on the totality of symptoms. Indeed, in many cases a remedy prescribed on the general and mental symptoms may greatly help a skin lesion. It may only be on further careful study of that remedy that skin symptoms are found to be present in the drug picture.

Local applications of Calendula ointment, simple cream, calamine, zinc and castor oil with a little coal tar may be needed to relieve cracking and itch, but these should be used sparingly. Steroid applications should be avoided whenever possible, as they have a suppressant rather than a curative action. Although valuable in certain acute situations they will never really cure the patient, and may inhibit the action of the homoeopathic remedy.

## GENERAL REMEDIES

**Antimonium Crudum**
Horny excrescences, callosities, corns, thickened tender soles of the feet.
Nails split. Warts on hands. Redness and inflammation of the eyelids.
Sore corners of mouth. Child cannot bear to be touched – irritable, night terrors. Greedy, fat people, oversentimental. Nausea and gastric upset from overindulgence. Tongue milky white.

**Antimonium Tartaricum**
One of the best remedies for *pustular* eruptions, impetigo, chickenpox and smallpox.
Pale sickly face with sunken eyes, drowsy, cold sweat.
Intense nausea relieved by vomiting. Thirstless. Coarse, rattling respiration in bronchitis, pneumonia or left heart failure.

**Graphites**
These patients are often obese, chilly, pale women, with a tendency to be lazy. They may blush easily or have nose bleeding. They are usually sad, despondent and weepy; apprehensive, timid and indecisive – music makes them weep.

*Skin* symptoms mainly affecting ears, hands and nails, mucous outlets, eyelids, corners of the mouth. Hard cracked skin or itchy, moist eruptions.

The nails are thick and out of shape. Cicatrices and scars may be helped by this remedy.

Scaliness and itching of the scalp.

There is crusting, blepharitis, and cracks behind the ears. The eruptions ooze a *thick honey-like fluid*. There may be a 'cobweb' sensation on the face.

Itchy, moist eruptions on scrotum.

### Mezereum

Itching eruptions worse from warmth of fire, at night.

Thick leather-like crust on the scalp with pus beneath.

The burning and itching of the eruptions is violent – must scratch.

Neuralgic pains also violent, especially in the face and jaw and following herpes zoster.

Twitchings of muscles and eyelids.

Craves fat ham.

Constant desire to eat.

Despondent and hypochondriacal from the pain or eruption.

### Petroleum

Patient is hot but skin feels cold in spots.

*Skin* symptoms are cracked, fissured palms or tips of fingers, with bleeding eruptions and *thin watery oozing*. Groin eruptions, worse in *winter*.

Redness, inflammation of the eyes with cracks on the lids and great itching. Chilblains, painful itching worse in cold weather.

Vesicles which break and form yellow crusts; itchy, burning vesicles of the genitals. (Rhus Tox.)

Occipital headache, vertigo, nausea worse in a boat or car. (A great seasickness remedy.)

Pains in stomach better from eating.

Diarrhoea preceded by colic – in the daytime.

### Psorinum

Sometimes regarded as a chilly Sulphur.

Rough, dry, cracking skin which looks dirty, rawness, itching and bleeding worse from bathing, worse from warmth of bed.

The patient is very *chilly* but the skin wants air.

*Offensive* discharges and eruptions with watery oozing.

Hair is dry and lustreless.

These patients lack vital reaction, are cold yet with night sweats. They are mentally despairing and hopeless.

### Rhus Tox.

Vesicular eruptions, burning, itching, sometimes pustular and like erysipelas.

Inflammation of the eyelids, with swelling and agglutination.

Blistering eruptions may occur on any part of the body, especially the genital area.

A good shingles remedy.

*Restlessness* – never at ease, must move.

Characteristic rheumatic pains worse from cold and wet, better from movement.

### Sulphur

This is one of the commonest and most valuable skin remedies.

The eruptions are characteristically burning and itching, with redness.

The body orifices are red – lips, nose, ears, anus, often with excoriating discharge. The eyelids are often red, with blepharitis. Septic lesions and boils are frequent. The skin lesions are aggravated by heat and after washing.

These patients are either lean, lank and philosophical, or stout with high colour, redness of the face and coarse hair. They are usually untidy and dislike washing, but do not be put off by a tidy Sulphur, where other symptoms fit.

General aggravation from heat and bath, with hot feet.

They usually feel empty mid-morning, and have a liking for sweet and tasty food and particularly fat and butter.

Morning diarrhoea occurs and the patient hates the smell of his stool, although not fussy in other ways.

### ACNE

This condition, predominantly found in adolescents, is sometimes most persistent, embarrassing and disfiguring. Tetracycline is still the mainstay in conventional treatment, and does improve some cases. Homoeopathy can also be of value.

### Calcarea Sulph.

This remedy is often of help given in 6c or 6x tablets twice daily over several weeks, and sometimes combined with a few doses of a high potency remedy suitable to the patient as a whole. The patient is usually cold, irritable and anxious about the future or his health. Headaches and bone pains better from heat.

Pimples and abscesses, burning and itching.
Offensive discharge from ears. Also useful in ischiorectal abscesses.

### Hepar Sulphuris
A lot of sepsis, inflamed, tender, better from local heat.
Chilly, sensitive to draughts, sour sweats.

### Kali Brom.
The bromine element, as one would expect, makes it useful in acne.
Fat, fair, lethargic, depressed, sleepy. Restless feet. Worry about themselves – not getting on well at school. Sensitive in case they are backward.
Coarse skin. *Severe acne* worse before menses. 2 a.m. itching.
Hot, aggravation heat and summer.

Sulphur, Silica and Natrum Mur. (with its greasy skin and eruption along the hair margin) may all be indicated depending on the patient's general symptoms.
Let me reiterate that any of the well-known, polycrest remedies may be required to deal with a skin condition, always prescribing for the patient as a whole, and not just for the local manifestations of his disease.

## BOILS AND ABSCESSES

### Hepar Sulph.
Inflamed, very sensitive, septic lesions, better from local heat, worse from pressure. The patient is oversensitive mentally and physically, irritable and even violent. Give the 10M potency 2 hourly until relief.

### Silica
A more chronic septic lesion. This remedy helps abscesses to discharge, and promotes suppuration and discharge of splinters and foreign bodies. The patient is chilly and sweaty.

### Sulphur
Recurring spots and septic lesions, often associated with skin eruptions, with heat and itching, aggravated by heat, in a hot hungry patient.

### Tarentula Cubensis
Carbuncles, large abscesses with several heads, burning and bluish in appearance.

*Dosage*
All these remedies should be given in 30c or higher potency and repeated 2 or 4 hourly for several doses, depending on severity.

## SHINGLES

**Arsenicum Album**
Burning eruption better from local heat.
Chilliness, restlessness, anxiety, midnight aggravation.

**Lachesis**
Bluish eruption, often left-sided, very sensitive to touch, better from
 local cold.
Hot patient with palpitations, choking, loquacity.

**Mezereum**
Already mentioned (see page 117).

**Ranunculus Bulbosus**
Frequently used in herpes zoster.
Stitching intercostal pains with great sensitivity, in both herpes and rheumatic conditions, pleurodynia aggravated by cold air, touch. Blue or transparent blisters which burn and leak serum, either round the chest wall or in supraorbital region.

**Rhus Tox.**
Vesicular eruptions, great restlessness, burning, itching, must scratch.

**Variolinum** (the smallpox nosode)
May be of help in postherpetic neuralgia.

# Chapter 17

# *Rheumatic and Arthritic Remedies*

This group of illnesses accounts for a large amount of disability and loss of working days. It includes a wide variety of ailments from simple muscular rheumatism to severe arthritis, and covers some neuralgic conditions and diseases like gout, polymyalgia rheumatica, systemic lupus erythematosus, psoriatic arthritis and connective tissue disorders.

It is important if possible to make an accurate diagnosis from the point of view of prognosis, and occasionally to select a steroid for a condition like temporal arteritis, with its risk of blindness. Apart from this, the homoeopathic physician must look again at the patient as a whole, with emphasis on causative factors, onset of illness, and the patient's general make-up and emotional reactions, as well as modalities of the local pain.

Sometimes the patient is so preoccupied by his pain and disability that it is difficult to see an overall picture. We may have to palliate with more local remedies initially, until a broad deep-acting remedy can be seen clearly. Conditions with gross pathological change such as severe rheumatoid arthritis we cannot expect to reverse, but we can still sometimes arrest the process and improve mobility and quality of life. Surgery now plays an important part in some of these.

Analgesics and antirheumatic drugs may be necessary to alleviate pain, but they have their own problems of allergy and toxicity. The minimum should be used to allow a clear prescribing picture to emerge, so that a more curative remedy may be found.

Certain modalities can be quite a help in selecting a remedy.

**Rheumatism**
Worse from warmth: Bryonia, Ledum, Phosphorus, Phytolacca, Pulsatilla, Thuja.
Better in cool: Ledum, Pulsatilla.
Better in warmth: Arsenicum, Causticum, Colchicum, Colocynth, Lycopodium, Mercurius, Nux Vomica, Rhus Tox., Sulphur.
Worse in dry cold: Aconite, Bryonia, Causticum, Hepar Sulph, Nux Vomica.

Worse in wet cold: Arnica, Colchicum, Dulcamara, Rhus Tox., Veratrum, Natrum Sulph.

Better from motion: Chamomilla, Dulcamara, Rhododendron, Rhus Tox., Pulsatilla.

This chapter contains some of the commonest rheumatic remedies. There are others, and in many cases a polycrest or constitutional remedy will have a more lasting effect.

### Bryonia

In contrast to Rhus Tox., Bryonia symptoms are *aggravated by movement*. This applies not only to joints, but also to headache, and pleural and chest pains. It affects muscles, fibrous tissues and synovia of joints with pain, redness, heat and swelling of effusion, all the symptoms being aggravated by any movement, and relieved by *pressure*, and often by cold. In acute rheumatism there is a heavy sour perspiration.

Other features of Bryonia are dryness of mucous membranes, lips, tongue, mouth, with thirst for large quantities at long intervals, aggravation in dry cold, east winds, and dislike of being disturbed, irritable and resentful of interference. Despondency and despair of recovery are often present.

### Colchicum Autumnale

This plant flowers in the autumn, and also has its characteristic symptoms, diarrhoea and rheumatism, in the autumn. It is known for its use in gout, but it has a wider field of action, and often Ledum is more indicated in gout.

The rheumatic *pains* of Colchicum move from joint to joint, are very sensitive to touch or motion. It affects small joints mainly, and the pain is worse in cold, damp weather, especially in the autumn, and better from heat and wrapping up.

This remedy has certain other symptoms which lead one to think of it. An intense *nausea* at the sight, smell or thought of food, burning and icy coldness in the stomach, and marked tympanitic distension of the abdomen with mucous diarrhoea.

The patients are very chilly and extremely irritable, and oversensitive to external impressions – the pain is unbearable (Chamomilla).

### Ferrum Metallicum

Often indicated in obese, chilly patients, who flush easily on excitement. The pains are worse when the limb is at rest and better from *slow* motion (like Pulsatilla), aggravated by rapid motion and better from heat.

The region most affected is the deltoid muscle and the shoulder.

These patients are often anaemic and tired, and have a marked aversion to eggs, with a tendency to vomit at night.

## Guaiacum

Chronic rheumatic conditions and gout, with weakness, emaciation and exhaustion, and sometimes associated with putrid expectoration found in bronchiectasis or tuberculosis.

Stitching, burning and neuralgic pains *worse* from *motion* and from *heat*.

Pains in the left side of the neck or on one side of the face, in the right shoulder, upper arm and chest muscles. Tearing pains in the right forearm and wrist, the *right thumb* and finger joints, again worse from *heat* and *motion*. Stitching pains around the knees and lower legs with shortening of the hamstrings. Swollen sensation in the limbs with bone pains.

The patient is thirsty with aversion to food, hot hands and night sweats.

## Kalmia

Affects muscles, tendons, joints and nerves. It is particularly useful where rheumatic complaints are related to previous syphilitic infections, or where cardiac complications have resulted from acute rheumatic fever.

The pains shoot and tear; they change about, wandering down the limbs from shoulder to fingers, or hips to toes, although they tend to go from lower limbs to upper limbs. Motion aggravates the pains, and can also cause vertigo.

Bone pains coming on in the night (like Syphilinum), as if the periosteum was torn off.

Neuralgia of the face, or post-herpetic neuralgia, stitching, tearing, cutting and shooting, coming on suddenly and then disappearing equally quickly.

Valvular heart disease of rheumatic origin, with slow pulse, palpitation worse lying on the left side, better lying on the back, when sitting up or bending forward.

## Ledum

*Chilly* person, but pains are characteristically relieved by *cold*.

A remedy for bruising, especially around the eye.

Rheumatic pains tend to begin in the lower limbs and ascend. The right hip and left shoulder are frequently involved and it is indicated in pains of the feet and ankles.

Swellings of joints are *pale*.

Gouty states and hard nodosities.

Stiffness of the joints and pain is better from cold and cold applications; worse from warmth of bed at night; worse from motion.

A remedy for puncture wounds. Wounds, abscesses and septic foci are tender but cold and *relieved by cold*, while those of Arsenicum burn, and are relieved by heat. Mottled, puffy, bloated face but cold. (Lachesis hot.)

## Phytolacca

Like Mercurius in its throat and mouth symptoms. The rheumatic pains are burning and shooting like electric shocks, worse on motion and during the night, on cold days and in cold damp weather, but worse from the heat of the bed. There is desire to move, but motion aggravates. Inflammation of fibrous sheaths. Pains particularly in the deltoid attachment and right shoulder joint, with stiffness and aching along the trapezius. Periarticular rheumatism in the temporo-mandibular joint. Stiff neck with pain on the slightest movement (where Bryonia and Rhus Tox. have failed to help).

A remedy of value in throat infections and in mastitis.

## Rhododendron

The rheumatic pains of this remedy are worse in cold, damp weather, windy weather and *thunderstorm*. The patient is generally upset in thundery or stormy weather. Pains are relieved *immediately* on moving, whereas in Rhus Tox. they are first sore and then improved by continued movement. They are better from warmth.

Tearing pains in the neck and back, driving him out of bed.
Pain in the shoulder joint so severe that the arm cannot be moved, relieved by walking about.
Rheumatic headache worse before a storm, better from wrapping up the head.
Neuralgia of the face and teeth.
Also of value in orchitis. (Pulsatilla too.)

## Rhus Toxicodendron

This remedy is one of the most commonly used in rheumatic conditions. It is characterised by aching pains and stiffness in almost any part of the body, in muscle and tendon, but also joints. The pains often come on after overexertion and particularly in damp, cold weather.

Pains and stiffness on *first moving* but *relieved by continued movement*, until the patient tires and must rest. They soon begin to ache again, become restless and start to move once more. Pain is better from heat and exercise. Restlessness and aggravated at night.

This remedy also has a characteristic vesicular skin eruption.

## Ruta

A remedy of injury and sprains – it particularly involves the periosteum and attachments of muscles and tendons, especially at wrists and ankles.

Sensations of weariness, as from a strain, or a fall or a blow, as if bruised.
Worse from cold and wet, and relieved by motion (like Rhus Tox.)
Its other spheres of action are in the eye, where it helps weak eye muscles or tired eyes, with poor accommodation (not the inflammation of Argentum Nit.), and in the rectum, where it is of value in weakness of muscle and prolapse of the rectum.
Helpful in osteoarthritis which follows an old sprain of the ankle or knee.

## Sanguinaria

A remedy of great value in sick headaches, where the pain extends from the occiput over the head to the right eye, and is accompanied by a bursting feeling and whizzing in the ears, followed by nausea and vomiting. Worse from sunrise until evening. The rheumatic pains are often in the *right* arm and shoulder, worse at night or turning in bed. Cannot raise the arm. Feeling of lassitude and weakness, not disposed to move or make any mental exertion. Worse in damp weather.

Also a useful remedy in chest conditions with badly smelling sputum, and tickling, hacking cough.

## Spigelia

This remedy is especially known for its pains. Hardly a nerve in the body escapes – shooting, burning, tearing, neuralgic pains, particularly in the *eyes, face, neck and shoulders*.

The pains in the eyes are relieved by cold, but all others are better from heat; any movement or jar aggravates.

Mention has already been made of its headaches, shooting over the left eye. Stabbing and neuralgic pains in the eyes, radiating in all directions, with tender eyeballs and disturbances of accommodation.

Stitching pains in the chest from intercostal neuralgia.

In chronic rheumatic diseases like rheumatoid and osteoarthritis it will often be necessary to seek a broad acting remedy for the patient as a whole. We must then study remedies like Kali Carb., Pulsatilla, Sulphur, Phosphorus, Natrum Mur., Calcarea Carb., Lycopodium, Sepia, Silica, Thuja and, of course, nosodes, particularly Medorrhinum and Tuberculinum.

# Chapter 18

# *Remedies of Depression and Anxiety*

In homoeopathy a great many commonly used remedies have strong mental symptoms, and the reader should study these as part of the total remedy picture described in Section III and in larger Materia Medicas. Also useful is Margaret Tyler's *Pointers to the Common Remedies, Number 6*, in which a large number of remedies are described for use in depression, grief, suicide, insane states, delusions, restlessness, excitement and violence, in loquacity, jealousy and suspicion.

It is important in mentally disturbed patients to elicit physical symptoms, generals, food cravings or aversions, and changes in the mental state from the normal for that patient. (For example, where a normally gentle, affectionate person becomes irritable, violent or suspicious, or an extrovert, friendly person becomes withdrawn, resentful and uncommunicative.) These changes from the normal will often indicate a remedy.

In severe psychotic states and schizophrenia it may be wise to seek psychiatric help, or have the patient admitted to a psychiatric unit for their own safety, or that of others.

There are, however, a large number of patients suffering from varying degrees of anxiety and depression who can be helped by homoeopathic remedies, thus reducing or even stopping their conventional tranquillisers and antidepressants, large quantities of which are now prescribed, often with little thought. In taking a patient's history, even for a physical complaint, we often find underlying disturbances of emotion due to past illness, family and social problems, resentments, anger, grief or fright. A quiet, careful history will often allow the doctor to help the patient to a better understanding of his or her symptoms, and advice may be all that is required. However a homoeopathic remedy covering as much as possible of the symptom picture may make a dramatic improvement in the patient's feeling of well being and ability to cope.

Polycrest remedies will often work best. We must observe the *indifference*, particularly to loved ones, of Sepia, Phosphorus and Phosphoric Acid; the marked *irritability* of remedies like Chamomilla and Nux Vomica; the *resentment* so characteristic of Natrum Mur. or

Staphisagria; the *lack of confidence* and *anxiety* of Silica or Lycopodium; the *fears* and emotions of Pulsatilla and Phosphorus; the *despair* of Aurum, Psorinum and Natrum Sulph.; and the effects of *fright* of Aconite and Opium; or *grief* of Ignatia and Natrum Mur. Study these broad-acting remedies in Section III and in larger Materia Medicas to understand the 'essence of feeling' of the remedy in its totality.

## DEPRESSION

### Aurum Metallicum
Suicidal depression with lack of confidence and irritability and anger from contradiction. Sulky, indisposed to talk, sits apart weeping and meditates on death. Full of self-condemnation but critical of others. Hysteria alternates with the depression, and there is apprehensive fear and terrifying dreams. Discontented with his circumstances and quarrelsome.

Prefers the open air and likes cool applications, but icy cold hands and feet.

### Calcarea Carbonica
Sometimes considered a slow, sluggish type of patient, but it has all sorts of *fears* in its symptomatology.

Despairs of life, imagines she will die, great uneasiness as if some accident or misfortune will happen.

Dread and anxiety for the future.

Fears of disease or death, that she will lose her reason, that people will observe her confusion, and that they look at her suspiciously.

Easily frightened, especially children, with night terrors and bad dreams.

Sits and fidgets with small things, and broods over things which are unimportant. Obstinate and peevish.

And of course the pale, flabby, sweaty person with cold extremities and sour vomit and stools.

### Cimicifuga (Actea Racemosa)
Especially a remedy for women with rheumatic and hysterical symptoms. Depression, anxiety and fear. The fear of death is almost as marked as in Aconite.

Depression is characterised by an awful *gloom*, like a black cloud, and yet mixed with hysterical symptoms and fears of the nature or extent of her illness. *Insomnia* in this type of person. A loquacious, suspicious temperament, will not take medicine in case there is something wrong with it (similar to Lachesis), and like this remedy, valuable in the menopause. A restless, irritable patient, gloomy but voluble, with flushes frequently colouring a pale face with dark rings under the eyes. Also a remedy with symptoms related to the generative organs, with painful, irregular menstruation, dysmenorrhoea *during* the flow and left ovarian pain. Mental disturbances in the puerperium, and therefore of value in post-partum depression. (Consider Sepia too, with its loss of interest in loved ones.)

Sensitive; to *cold* and damp, with rheumatic pains, which are better when the mental symptoms are worse.

*Headaches* especially in the nape of the neck, and with pain behind the eyes, relieved by cool open air, and worse from movement.

### Drosera

This remedy is predominantly thought of for whooping cough, but it is also a remedy to think of where there is a history of tuberculosis, and it has marked mental symptoms in its picture.

Dejected over what others have done to him. Disheartened and concerned about the future. Imagines he has been deceived by spiteful, envious people. Resentful of insults, can become quite enraged over trifles.

Anxiety marked especially in the evening, with desire to end his life by drowning. Dreams of being maltreated. Restless, cannot stick at one thing for any length of time.

### Natrum Sulphuricum

A useful remedy where there is a history of head injury, or in patients with asthma or pneumonia, particularly involving the left base of the lung, and occurring in warm wet weather.

Depressed, tearful, with a tendency to weep or feel sad from music (Graphites also). Tired of life but does not really want to end it (Aurum does).

Irritable in the mornings, hates to speak or be spoken to, sensitive to the smallest noise.

4–5 a.m. aggravation.

### Phosphoric Acid

The key characteristic of this remedy is its remarkable *indifference* to everything. He does not want anything, does not want to speak, shows no interest in the outside world, cannot collect his thoughts properly. Listless and apathetic.

Ailments from care, grief, chagrin, homesickness or disappointed love, but *without* the sensitivity, hysteria or changes of mood of Ignatia, *without* the intensity and tendency to go to pieces on account of chagrin or resentment seen in Staphisagria. Natrum Mur. is far more intense and passionate, weeps and hates sympathy, whereas Phosphoric Acid has dull apathy in its disappointed love.

Overgrown, overweight children, with growing pains and headaches.

In spite of the prostration running through this remedy there is one contradiction, in that the profuse diarrhoea often seen in Phosphoric Acid does not cause exhaustion, and indeed the patient may feel better after diarrhoea. (Calcarea Carb. better when constipated.)

## Psorinum

This remedy is thought of most often in skin diseases, but it has profound mental symptoms.

A very chilly remedy, with foulness of discharges.

Hopelessness, despair of recovery and fears he will die. Full of fears and forebodings, that he will fail in his business. Dreams of his business.

## RESTLESSNESS, VIOLENCE AND DELIRIUM

### Arsenicum Album

No group of restless remedies can omit Arsenicum.

*Restlessness* is a constant symptom, accompanied by *prostration* out of all proportion to the symptoms. *Anxiety* about himself – full of fear, feels it is useless to take medicine as he is sure to die. Extremely fastidious, and sensitive to smells, touch and surroundings.

Together with the chilliness, burnings, and aggravation of symptoms at 1–2 a.m. described elsewhere.

Nash describes Belladonna, Hyoscyamus and Stramonium as remedies particularly indicated in delirium.

### Belladonna

This remedy is one of our commonest acute remedies, and has been mentioned in fever, inflammation and headache.

The patient is hot, flushed and dry, with dilated pupils and very dry red throat with constant desire to swallow. *Sudden* onset of symptoms with violence. The child with a high fever has delirium, nightmares, sees animals and ghosts, but the fears and violence are also seen in mentally disturbed patients. There is congestive headache, and the patient is frightened and wants to run away and hide.

### Hyoscyamus

Here the patient is pale and weak, often elderly, and the lowgrade type of delirium predominates with muttering stuporose state, staring at surrounding objects without seeing them, picking at the bedclothes. Now and then violent outbursts occur and the patient becomes restless, getting out of bed and taking off his clothes or talking and singing amorously. This picture is seen in pneumonia and typhoid states, but also in elderly patients who are confused and in strange surroundings, like a hospital. They are often very suspicious, imagining that the nurse is trying to poison them, and refusing their medicine. They are also jealous of others (these last two symptoms being seen in Lachesis also). Twitchings of muscles occur all over the body, particularly in the stuporose state.

## Stramonium

This is the wildest of these three delirious remedies. It resembles Belladonna in the redness of the face and dilated pupils, but above all these patients are *loquacious*. Raving, singing, laughing, swearing or praying. Repeatedly jerking the head up from the pillow, or throwing himself about. Fears being alone and in the dark.

# Chapter 19

# *Remedies in the Elderly*

In homoeopathy there are no remedies exclusively for use in the elderly, because any patient may need almost any remedy depending on the total symptom picture, and to some extent the pathology of the condition. Again polycrest remedies will often be indicated, and should always be considered first, but there are some which should be borne in mind for the old and which are easily forgotten.

Potencies can be varied as with other age groups, but it should be remembered that a weak, elderly patient may not have the ability to respond to very high potencies, and may do better on 30c. Some patients with a lot of pathological change may require 6x or 3x potencies given over quite a long period to alleviate rather than to cure, where this is not possible. However, many old people live an active and alert life to a great age, helped by their homoeopathic remedies. We are now very aware of the care required in giving orthodox drugs to the old, who often react very badly to sedatives, antibiotics, antihypertensives, and certain cardiac remedies, and are better with only small doses, or in many cases no drugs at all. We have no problem such as this with homoeopathic treatment, which is gentle and safe in its action.

A few remedies for the old or those with loss of memory or confusion are considered in this section.

## Ambra Grisea

Premature old age. Feeble, trembling, tottering of gait, a dreamy state with forgetfulness. Jumps from one subject to another, asking questions but not waiting for the answer before moving on to another. Alternation of depression with vehemence of temper. Has to make an unusual effort to bring his mind back to concentrate on what he was thinking about. His mind dwells on most disagreeable things and he cannot get rid of them. Vertigo in old men, so bad that he cannot go out in the street. Symptoms all worse in the mornings. The presence of others aggravates symptoms – this is noticeable in old people who cannot pass a stool in the presence of a nurse or relation, and are often constipated. Also aggravation from conversation, and music seems to be intolerable. Itching in old people.

## Anacardium Orientale

This remedy is of value where there is loss of memory, especially in the elderly, but it has a characteristic sensation of dual personality, as if he has two wills in conflict. Everything seems in a dream; has a marked inferiority and worry over his forgetfulness. This applies also to younger patients like students, with fear of failure and anticipation of the ordeal of examinations.

Along with the memory loss there is irritability and desire to curse and swear, sometimes in those with a strict sense of morality or religious faith. This distresses them greatly and causes feelings of guilt. Can be quite malicious. Sensations of a plug in the rectum or the ear, or of a band or hoop round a part.

Dyspepsia and pain in the stomach when it is empty, and relieved by eating.

## Arnica

This remedy is almost specific for injury or bruising, but it is of value in severe illness or in elderly patients. Old people who get easily tired, or do too much and feel exhausted, will often benefit from a dose of Arnica.

Great weariness and a sensation *as if bruised* is a key indication. This may follow overexertion or a fall, but also occurs in patients who are in bed a lot or seriously ill, perhaps with cancer. The bed feels hard – he is sore and restless and helped by change of position. (The Arsenicum patient is restless, but anxious and frightened, and not helped by moving; the Rhus Tox. patient must move and is relieved by moving.)

A very *ill* patient may say he *feels well*.

Coldness of the body with hot head.

Irritable, sad, hopeless, indifferent. Does not want to be touched – because of pain; very sensitive even to the approach of a nurse.

Dreadful dreams and imaginings – reliving the events of an accident. Horror of instant death.

## Baryta Carbonica

A remedy for slow development in children, but also in degenerative, cardiovascular or cerebral conditions of old age. Enlarged glands and prostatic hypertrophy.

Chilly, pale, withered with weakness.

Premature old age, childish behaviour in the elderly, not clear in his intellect, memory loss, cannot think clearly.

Fear of something going to happen. Hatches up all sorts of complaints and grievances, imaginary worries. Thinking of his troubles makes him worse.

Coarse catarrhal rattling in the chest in old age, particularly in cold, winter weather (Senega, Ammoniacum).

## Carbo Vegetabilis

We think of this remedy in faint and collapse, where the patient is cold, pale, sweaty with thready pulse and a desire for air (in heart cases or post-operative collapse). It is also of great value as an old person's remedy, a dose of 30c given at regular intervals or 6x tablets twice daily.

There is slowness, sluggishness and indifference.

Internal burning sensations but coldness externally, especially feet and legs, hands and nose. Venous sluggishness, blueness, varicose conditions. Much flatulence.

## Cocculus

A remedy useful where the patient suffers from the effects of loss of sleep, coupled with anxiety as in nursing a loved one. She is weak, prostrated, cannot sleep or suffers anxious, frightful dreams. There is congestive headache, and vertigo with nausea, with extreme sensitivity to motion. This may occur in Menière's syndrome, cerebral ischaemia or even in travel sickness. There is overwhelming nausea at the thought or smell of food.

Paralytic stiffness of limbs, weakness of the back and legs, of the neck muscles, and numbness of feet and hands. Paralysis of eyelids and throat, and inco-ordination like Gelsemium. Anxious, melancholy, sensitive to insults or disappointment, slow concentration or in answering, cannot find the right word, cannot bear noise or contradiction.

## Conium

Progressive weakness of memory, mind becomes tired and he cannot concentrate or stand any mental effort. He is unhappy, indifferent to things, peevish and will sit and mope in a corner. Any kind of excitement brings on physical or mental distress. Useful in widows or widowers denied a sexual outlet, and who become hysterical or hypochondriac as a result of this.

Vertigo on turning the head, worse when lying down, worse on moving the eyes and better if the eyes are closed.

Trembling and paralytic symptoms, and a curious symptom where aching in the legs from rheumatism or ulceration is better from allowing the legs to hang down.

# Chapter 20

# *Children's Remedies*

While there are certain illnesses more commonly encountered in children in general practice, the basic principles of homoeopathic prescribing remain the same – to seek a remedy most suitable to the child as a whole, and having symptoms most similar in its 'drug picture' to those presenting in the patient. In using homoeopathic remedies we can give the same quantity in the same potency at the same intervals, whatever the age, from the newborn to the very elderly. In acute illness 30c or 10M are most frequently prescribed, and in more chronic conditions, a few doses of 30c will again prove satisfactory.

We believe that a homoeopathic remedy acts in a very small dose because the effect depends on a selective action for that individual, at that particular time, and because an ill person is sensitive to a small dose which would not affect a healthy person. For that reason, a large quantity of a single potentised remedy, or a mixture of remedies taken at one time, will not cause a reaction (whereas repeated doses of a single remedy for some days or weeks may cause the effect of a proving, with aggravation of symptoms). Hence if a child inadvertently finds your medicine case, and swallows the contents of several bottles at once, no untoward effects will result and nothing need be done.

## ACUTE CONDITIONS

The commonest ones seen in children are injuries, infectious fevers, and acute respiratory and gastrointestinal complaints. Remedies for these are described in the relevant chapters of this section, the symptom pictures applying equally to adults and children. Here a good knowledge of a few acute remedies like Aconitum, Arnica, Ferrum Phos., Belladonna, Arsenicum Alb., Chamomilla, Pulsatilla, Phosphorus and Sulphur will go a long way to helping most cases. They are safe and rapid in action with no side effects.

# CHRONIC CONDITIONS – BORLAND'S FIVE GROUPS

When you are faced with more chronic problems such as recurrent coughs and colds, allergies, eczema, asthma, bed-wetting, constipation or behaviour problems, try to look for the patient's remedy, a constitutional prescription for the child rather than his illness.

Dr D. M. Borland was one of the great observers of children, and in his book *Children's Types* he vividly portrays various kinds of children in groups, numbered 1 to 5, giving not only a picture of their symptoms and behaviour, but often comparing one remedy with another. These are by far the best children's studies available in our Materia Medica, and I make no apology for describing these in an abbreviated form in this chapter. This may help you initially in selecting a remedy and encourage you to read his comparisons, which aid you to distinguish one from another. Each of the five groups described contains a set of related remedies. The descriptions of the related remedies follow on naturally one after the other.

*Group One* is the Calcarea group: Calcarea Carb., Calcarea Phos., Phosphorus, Silica, Lycopodium, Causticum, Tuberculinum.

*Group Two* is the Baryta Carb. group: Baryta Carb., Borax, Natrum Mur., Sepia., Aurum, Carbo Veg.

*Group Three*, the Graphites group, contains remedies useful in skin conditions: Graphites, Capsicum, Psorinum, Antimonium Crudum and Petroleum.

*Group Four* is the Pulsatilla group, mostly hot blooded remedies: Pulsatilla, Sulphur, Thuja, Iodine, Fluoric Acid.

*Group Five*, the Arsenic group, contains nervous and emotional remedies: Arsenicum Alb., Chamomilla, Cina, Magnesia Carb., Ignatia, Zincum.


**Calcarea Carbonica (Group 1)**
Soft, smooth, smiling baby, with sweaty head. Fat, fair, chilly, lethargic. Lack of energy. Tendency to rickets, big head, slow closure of fontanelles. Although chilly they get hot on the slightest exertion, sweat at night, and may stick their feet out of bed (Pulsatilla, Sulphur, Chamomilla). Sluggish mentally and physically, slow at school and at games, weak muscles and ankles. Content to sit and do nothing, clumsy, give up easily, sensitive to criticism or being laughed at.

Scared, especially when unwell or alone, and of going to bed in the dark. Night terrors and dreams – seeing faces. Aggravation from physical or mental exertion, or rapid motion – car and train sick.

Dislike of too hot food, aversion to meat and craving for eggs, and often indigestible things – chalk, coal.

Constipation – but tend to be more comfortable this way – laxatives upset them. Stools often pale and diarrhoea if chilled.

Liable to catch colds, tonsils and glands enlarged. In children, this remedy can be given repeatedly, even although the child is improving.

## Calcarea Phosphorica (Group 1)

Here the child, while still retaining many of the Calcarea Carb. characteristics, is thinner, with adenoidal tissue and small cervical glands. Brighter at school and definitely growing, often with *pains* in the legs, particularly muscular pains.

*Headaches* in growing girls, when studying. Dislike of interference. The child is restless, moving about, reluctant to talk, discontented and peevish – always complaining that something is wrong. Indisposition to work, cannot concentrate. Full of vague fears and dreads, especially in the evening. Anxiety causes tummy upsets and diarrhoea – colic in infants after eating – green, slimy hot, watery stools. These children love *tasty* foods, ham rind, kippers. They are upset by ice-cream and cold drinks.

A useful remedy in recurring coughs and colds in growing children.

## Phosphorus (Group 1)

Slim, with either reddish hair and freckles, or brown hair and eyes and long eyelashes. (like Tuberculinum Bovinum).

*Chilly* except for head and stomach, which prefer cold.

Sweats, if anxious or on much exertion.

Liable to flush on excitement or with hot food.

Affectionate and like sympathy and attention, and physical touch, but not so much if very ill – indifference.

If tired or upset can fly into a passion.

*Fears* – dark, thunder, especially at twilight – sensitive to atmosphere.

Headache better in cold air, prefer to be propped up, and not lying flat. Hunger before headache.

Desire salty taste, sour, cold – *thirst* for large cold drinks.

Colds start with one blocked nostril, one running – bleeding.

Raw hacking cough worse lying on left side, worse going from hot to cold air, but prefer fresh air, worse on talking.

Right basal lung inflammation.

## Silica (Group 1)

*Chilly*, thin child, with fine hair, light brown. Pale, *sweaty* especially feet, and hands which are clammy – hands go dead, improved when put in hot water.

Tendency to sepsis, boils, septic cuts or eczema, poor nails.

Lack of strength, easily exhausted by talking and, therefore, dislikes speaking. Shy, lack of confidence, *dread of failure*, over conscientious, *resentful*, but can be witty and good fun if encouraged.

Likes cold food and drink; milk upsets; hot drink causes sweating.

Headaches: better from heat and wrapping up the head, worse from cold, physical or mental exertion.

## Lycopodium (Group 1)

Thin child, growing, sallow complexion and thicker skin than Phosphorus.

Chilly, but sensitive to stuffy atmosphere.

Desire for *sweet* foods and *hot* food or drink.

Liable to digestive upsets, good appetite but failure to gain weight. Enlarged abdomen, but not the palpable mesenteric glands of the Calcarea salts.

Headaches from overwork at school, like Calcarea Phos. – a dull ache.

Anxious, *diffident*, lacks assurance, tends to *worry* and become keyed up before events. Liable to bite his nails. Often the worried frown.

Right sided symptoms.

Aggravation between 4–8 p.m.

## Causticum (Group 1)

Sallow appearance, usually thin.

Rheumatic symptoms *better in damp weather*. May get acute muscular rheumatism, particularly from exposure to cold dry wind. Stiffness about the joints and growing pains.

Facial palsy or torticollis developing after exposure to an icy wind.

When overworked or nervously distressed they get chorea symptoms, with jerking persisting during sleep.

Clumsiness and liability to strain muscles (Calcarea – the ankles).

Aversion to sweet foods (opposite of Lycopodium).

*Acute thirst* after meals, when they have digestive upset.

*Sensitive* children – to pain and any emotional disturbance – the idea of pain is **worse** – if they think another child is being hurt, they will cry.

*Warts*

Nocturnal enuresis.

## Tuberculinum Bovinum (Group 1)

Particularly where there is a family history of tuberculosis. It is usually unwise to give this remedy when the child is actually suffering from tuberculosis in an acute phase.

'Tub' children are often like the Phosphorus child in appearance, slender, attractive with red lips, brown eyes and dark hair and long beautiful eyelashes. There is often a fine 'down' of hair running down the middle of the back.

A valuable remedy in children with repeated cough, colds or chest infections, usually given as a single dose, between other remedies like Calcarea Phos., Phosphorus, or Silica.

Periodicity of symptoms or intermittent fever.
Desire for salt, cold milk. Eats well but remains thin.
Temper tantrums in children. Love of change or travel.


### Baryta Carbonica (Group 2)

This is the main drug to consider in children who are *backward*. They also tend to be small for their age, late in speaking, walking, dentition, gaining weight.

Excessive *shyness*, nervous of strangers, of being left alone, of going out of doors and, in a town child, of going into open fields.
*Touchy*, don't like interference, easily irritated.
*Forgetful*, never play long with one toy, lack of attention and ability to concentrate – this is noticeable in the older child at school.
Any sustained effort exhausts them – they become irritable, and in older children this leads to frontal headache.
*Chilly* and liable to catch colds.
Recurring sore throats and hypertrophied tonsils, enlarged glands.

Also enlarged abdominal glands, poor posture, prominent abdomen. Eating aggravates – touchy, tired and irritable after eating. Constipation.

Crusty skin eruption on the head, crusty eyelids and general upset from washing. (Psorinum has these symptoms and follows well.) The skin eruption may be very irritable although there is not much to see on the surface.


### Borax (Group 2)

Pale, earthy, suffering expression.

May be similar to look at as Baryta Carb. and a bit slow mentally and perhaps under size, but *frightened*. *Fright* from noise (sudden) – child starts at slightest noise, and from pain. Night terrors but usually with some cause – child doing too much in the day, or overexcited in the evening – then night terror. Aggravation from *downward motion* – terror. (Lift, or baby being put down.)

Valuable in air sickness (dropping sensation and terror).
*Stomatitis* – Salivation with white spots on the tongue, lips or inside of the cheek.

Herpetic eruptions about the lips, or a generalised herpetic eruption on the body.

Mucous membrane inflammation may cause pain on micturition, without definite infection, and possibly enuresis.

*Mentals* – Inability to learn, from *idleness* – if they would put their hearts into it they could learn. Never settle to anything, even at play they won't stick to anything. Get bored and change from one thing to another.

Much more irritable than Baryta Carb. Irritability ends in passion – kicking and screaming.

*Stomach* – Acute attacks of diarrhoea and vomiting, particularly colic after fruit.

Borax child gets nausea and sickness from intense concentration; Baryta Carb. gets frontal headache.

### Natrum Muriaticum (Group 2)

These children are usually undersized and underweight. They appear shy but really more *resent interference* or being handled, and will burst into tears. They tend to cry more with *rage* than with terror (which the Baryta Carb. child does).

If they are crying, *firmness* helps to settle them, or allowing them just to sit in a corner and watch. Soothing makes them worse. Natrum Mur. children are awkward and knock things over, due to being in a hurry rather than clumsy. They are often slow in learning to speak, and may stammer or have faulty speech due to difficulty in articulation.

They tend to have thin necks and small, shotty glands at the back of the neck.

*Skin eruptions* occur at the margin of the hair; there is a greasy appearance of the face, and tendency to acne in teenagers. The tongue has red and white patches which are sensitive, like the mapped tongue in the adult. A tendency to herpes on the lips. The remedy again has pressing frontal headaches over the eyes, especially from study and mental concentration (like Baryta Carb. and Calcarea Phos.).

*Chilly* persons, sensitive to draughts, shivering or sneezing from change of temperature, but also very *sensitive to heat*, stuffiness and exposure to the sun, causing headache.

*Salt* craving.

Hang-nails, splits at the sides of nails, sensitive and slow to heal.

### Sepia (Group 2)

Sallow, greasy skin.

Depressed, moody, sluggish, disinclined to work and even loss of interest in playing. A *negative* attitude to everything. If pushed they will sulk or weep.

Nervous, scared of being alone, of the dark, and yet dislike of being

handled (Natrum Mur.). Dislike of going to parties or meeting friends, due to sluggishness, but once they get there they brighten up, and if they *dance* they come alive, and are happy (adults too).
Tendency to nod the head.
Constipation and associated enuresis, usually in the first sleep, before 10 p.m.
Tendency *to faint*, especially in a close atmosphere, standing at school or in church.
Sensitive to *cold* – develops a cold from any change of weather.
*Greedy* child, upset by milk.
Tendency to sweat; itching of skin without much eruption.

## Aurum (Group 2)
Sallow, dispirited, sluggish child – depressed negative attitude.
An undeveloped child –not necessarily small but slow in developing (like Baryta Carb.).
Often boys – undescended testicle.
Lifelessness, miserable and lacking in 'go', no initiative – everything seems an effort. Backward at school, poor memory, but if contradicted they fly into a rage.
In spite of sluggishness, they are terrified of pain and very sensitive to it. Sensitive to noise, and have acute sense of taste and smell.
Sensitive to disappointment – grieve for days; out of all proportion.
Sobbing in sleep, without waking and without distress the night before.
*Catarrh* persistent. Infected hypertrophied tonsils, with offensive secretion in the crypts.
Offensive nasal discharge.
Otitis media with tonsillitis and often purulent, smelly ear discharge.

## Carbo Vegetabilis (Group 2)
This remedy picture is not really a type in its own right, but develops as a *result* of a preceding illness, such as measles, bronchitis or pneumonia, influenza or whooping cough.
The child is *sluggish*, dull, lacking in 'go', easily discouraged, peevish, slow in reacting.
Also sluggish *circulation*, Heavy, sallow complexion with bluish fingers and toes, and coldness of the extremities.
Dull, *occipital headaches*, with inability to work or concentrate. When tired and having headaches he gets violent nightmares, of ghosts, faces.
Although cold and sluggish they are liable to get *hot* and *sweaty* at night, with sour smelling sweat, generalised, but particularly on the extremities.

Epistaxis.

*Digestive* upset, with flatulence, constipation and swollen abdomen.
Attacks of diarrhoea, offensive, watery in-between.
*Desire* for *sweet* things, which upset, and *salt*.
*Aversion* to *fat* and rich food, which upsets, and *milk*.


## Graphites (Group 3)

Fat, heavy pale child with large head, and droopy eyelids. Flabby with
muscular weakness, easily tired out, and sensitive to motion, travel.
Rheumatoid pains affect the neck and lower limbs.

*Chilly* – like to be covered up but prefer air. Unstable circulation.
When excited tend to flush up and even get epistaxis.

*Mentally* they are timid, miserable and lack assurance; they hesitate
in replying and cannot make decisions. Tend to be lazy and averse to
work. Although sluggish, lazy and uncertain, they are anxious. Tend to
look on the hopeless side, look for trouble, dread new school. Critical.
Sensitive to music which makes them weep.

*Skin* – most Graphites patients have some skin complaint. Harsh dry
skin (unlike the soft sweaty skin of Calcarea). Tendency for fingers to
crack and bleed on exposure to cold or in cold water.

Sticky, yellow oozing discharge. Cracks and discharge behind ears, at
corners of mouth and eyes, bends of elbows, groins.
Fissures at anus. Crusts form with gluey discharge underneath.
Chronic otitis with discharge, and the same sticky yellow discharge
causing eczema of the external ear.
Nasal discharge and large tonsils.
Blepharitis with sticky eyelids.
Adolescents get acute acne.
Big appetite, upset if empty, better from eating.
Dislike of *sweet* and *fish*.
Attacks of abdominal cramp relieved by hot milk.
*Constipation* – feels upset by it, worries over it. Stool may contain
stringy mucus.
Sleepy in day – slow to get to sleep.


## Capsicum (Cayenne or Red Pepper) (Group 3)

*Burnings.*
Fat, rather lazy, *obstinate* child with clumsy movements – rarely neat.
Flabby. Chilly.
Reddish cheeks, or pale and flush up like Graphites.
Sluggish, rather backward with chronic hoarseness and a history of
acute sore throats (not quinsies, but just acute throats), transitory
attacks of earache.

*Mentals* – Forgetful on an errand, partly due to lack of attention.

Touchy, easily offended, easily irritated. Strange dislike of being away from home – perhaps due to being touchy and lazy and a feeling that they are not appreciated. They have to make an effort, and can be agreeable when away – at home they may be unpleasant. Hypersensitive to noise, touch. Dull, slow at school, poor memory.

*Local hyperaemia* – in earache whole ear bright crimson. In rheumatism one joint affected and it has a localised blush over it.

Bright crimson face with enlarged tonsils, *burning heat* in the mouth and intense thirst. They want cold drinks during fever but this makes them shiver.

Sore throats with *beginnings of a mastoid*, often blowing up at night – restless, irritable, sleepless – blush over the mastoid and hyperaesthesia. Also valuable in *chronic ear discharge* with eczema of the external ear.

Capsicum children often have acute cystitis, *burning,* intense irritable pain on urination.

## Psorinum (Group 3)

Thin, sickly children, with lack of stamina, easily exhausted by any effort, physical or mental. Liable to become mentally confused under stress. Dispirited, hopeless, peevish and irritable.

They look unhealthy, *dirty* and unwashed.

Dry, rough skin, with tendency to smelly sweat.

*Skin lesions* like Graphites, but with a watery or purulent, offensive discharge. *Intense irritation*, worse from *washing*.

Scratches the skin till it bleeds, nearly driven distracted.

Acute blepharitis, purulent nasal discharge, excoriating the lip, and smelly otorrhoea.

Abnormal appetite; lack of food causes violent headache.

Useful in hayfever prophylaxis, a single dose in the spring, not in the acute phase.

## Antimonium Crudum (Group 3)

Overweight, fat, pale children with tendency to redness round the eyes, and moist eruption behind the ears.

Mentally, these children are a contradiction.

On the one hand irritable, peevish and made worse by soothing (Natrum Mur.). Night terrors.

On the other, impressionable, sensitive, easily upset emotionally, liable to burst into tears from emotional stress, or if their feelings are touched. Under stress they become pale and faint.

*Skin eruptions:* large, crusty, smelly eruptions – the typical crusty impetigo on the face.

Skin lesions are made much worse by washing (Sulphur, Psorinum), inflamed and painful from radiant heat.
Clumsy, jerky movements.
_Warts_ – numerous, flat, on fingers.
Deformed, thickened nails; also tender thick skin on soles.
_Digestive_ upset from acids, sour fruits or sour drinks.
Tongue soft, flabby and coated _white_.


## Petroleum (Group 3)

Again a remedy with skin eruptions, but a thin child with an abnormal appetite, even hungry between meals.

A _seasick_ and train-sick remedy, but often with occipital headache accompanying the nausea (which Tabacum does not have).

Irritable, _quarrelsome_, easily offended.
Mentally bright, but lazy, inattentive and forgetful at school.
Sensitive to _noise_, sudden or loud noise – scares them. Nervous of crowds.
_Chilly_ .
_Skin eruptions:_ deep, painful cracks with watery yellow fluid, behind ears, in folds, corners of mouth, anus, groins, axilla.
Sensitive crusts, tendency to bleed.
Itch is most marked in the day (Sulphur at night).
Cracks and _painful bleeding fissures_ on fingers.
Liable to _colds;_ nose blocked, excoriating discharge, crusts, deafness, otitis with watery discharge, redness and eczema of the ear.
Itchy eyes, blepharitis and lachrymal duct infection.
Bladder irritation, cystitis, raw and smarting; enuresis.
Abdominal colic and diarrhoea on exposure to cold – raw, red anus and perineum.


## Pulsatilla (Group 4)

There are two types of Pulsatilla child. One is small, finely built, with fine skin and hair, unstable circulation, liable to flush up from emotion and then go pale, shy, sensitive, affectionate, easy to handle and definitely responsive, bright and gay.

The other, less often remembered, is fatter, with more colour, rather darker hair, more sluggish in reaction, with more tendency to weep, craving for attention, but less responsive.

_Sensitive to heat_ – they flag, lose their energy and sparkle, hang about and get tearful or irritable.
Liable to _digestive upsets_ – particularly if _chilled or cold_ during a hot spell – they get sick or have diarrhoea, cystitis or earache.

Taking ice-cream in hot weather upsets – rich food upsets, like butter and cream, but dislike fat.

During fever they get *chilly*, shivery. Often acute colds with coryza, gastric upset, nausea or even vomit. Although chilly their head is better in the open air, worse in a *stuffy room* and there is *bland* nasal discharge.

*Conjunctivitis* – eyes stream in the open air, sensitive to cold draught, photophobia, itching of eyelids and styes on the lower lid.

*Earache* – usually from exposure to cold; violent pain spreading over the face, bursting feeling, better from *cold* applications.

*Sunset* aggravation, nervous with tendency to *nightmares*, fear of the dark and being left alone, yet most lively in the evening and before bed.

Giddiness from looking up at high things.

Sleeps with hands above his head.

### Sulphur (Group 4)

There are two types of Sulphur child. The first is of a heavier build, coarse hair, big head, high colour with rough skin and red extremities, hands and feet. Also redness of lips and ears and eyelids, with blepharitis and styes.

The second is thin, with big head and spindly legs, biggish abdomen, paler colour and rough skin, dry with tendency to split or crack. A miserable, seedy child, easily tired, liable to weep and attempts to comfort annoy him. Inability to stand long, irritable if hungry.

Heavier Sulphurs are quarrelsome, impatient, critical, fault finding and discontented, and lazy, possibly due to tiredness on exertion.

Dislike of interference.

Sluggish, dull and cross, and yet when stimulated *they can* be *bright* and *interesting, friendly* and often clever.

Pleased with their possessions; toys, family, car are all better than others.

*Skin irritation* – worse in warm and at night. Pleasurable sensation from scratching. Every kind of eruption, intense irritation of all kinds.

*Redness* of orifices, nose, ears, mouth, urethra, anus.

*Heat aggravates* but unstable mechanism – waves of heat and chilliness.

Sometimes hot head and cold hands, or hot hands and cold feet – not all Sulphurs have hot feet. Bathing aggravates. They smell – eruptions, discharges, perspiration.

*Desire tasty*, highly seasoned foods, also sweet. Food that is out of the ordinary. Sluggish and sleepy after meals.

Upset by milk, may get diarrhoea. Some children, like adults, like fat.

Usually constipated with big abdomen.

Terrifying nightmares.

Chronic nasal discharges – offensive, excoriating.

Chronic tonsillitis, infected, hot, offensive breath, masses of glands. Shivering, sweating and thirst in attacks.

Chronic ear discharges, excoriating, pain aggravated by hot applications.

Chest conditions – chilly in a draught, but cannot stand stuffy atmosphere.

Jaundice in children.

Rheumatism, with sweat, heat, red tongue worse from heat, better from movement.

### Thuja (Group 4)

The Thuja child tends to be small and finely built, dark or fair. He may be slightly backward, but sometimes the lively, active child gives this impression because he hesitates and finds difficulty in choosing or saying words, and this makes him appear slow.

Disinclined to talk, rather silent. Activity seems to brighten them up, but they become dull and heavy if left to sit.

Extremely sensitive, responds to kindness, is easily upset emotionally, conscientious, and in particular *sensitive* to *music* – may even weep from music. Sad and may weep like Pulsatilla.

Sensitive to the *cold* and damp but better in the open air. Worse in the mornings.

Greasy skin, especially in dark children. Fair children may have down on the back, like Tuberculinum Bovinum.

Sweating on exertion and *sweat* on *being uncovered.*

Neuralgic *headaches* on mental stress, or when overtired or overexcited. These pains may be in localised areas, which are painful and sensitive.

Chronic *catarrh*– thick yellowish green – crusts in nose, chronic otitis media.

Poor *digestion* – particularly upset by onions and in older children by tea.

Gurgling in the abdomen, full boggy caecum with attacks of diarrhoea. Pale, greasy almost fatty stools with flatus.

*Warts* – soft, tend to bleed.

Upset from vaccination.

### Iodine (Group 4)

Dark haired, dark skinned, thin. A bit like the Sulphur child, but without skin problems.

Intense restlessness – fidgeting.

Sensitive to *heat* – room, bath, sun.

*Irritability* – sudden, impulsive – may strike another, although playing quite happily. Following this they get depressed and silent and lose interest.

*Hunger* – exhausted if long without a meal, headaches.

Although they eat, they don't gain weight.

Acute nose infection, hot, watery, irritant discharge, sinus pain, sneezing, watering eyes, but nose feels obstructed.

Chronic eustachian catarrh and deafness.

With the cold they get laryngitis, hoarse, painful, croup.

Intensely hot dry skin with croup – restless, anxious, like Arsenic but it is chilly and perspires a bit – Iodine is hot and dry.

Asthmatic breathing, better in open air.

Diarrhoea attacks – frothy, fatty, whitish stools, perhaps pancreatic in origin.

In children with bright red cheeks you may get acute rheumatism – violent pains better on moving, worse from heat, sharp and stabbing.

Like Bryonia but it is thirsty, white tongue, more dull and heavy and averse to food. (Iodine – alert, hungry.)


## Fluoric Acid (Group 4)

Often fair-haired, thin, fine boned, a bit like Silica to look at. Sensitive to *heat* – hot room, hot sun, too many clothes. Red sweaty palms, offensive foot sweat but hot and sore. Unhealthy finger nails, brittle, cracked, splintered. Dry and fissured tongue.

*Mentals* – Yielding disposition, but not very irritable, patient, and enjoyment of life – of the simplest things, cheerful.

Tired with mental concentration, headaches at school and not very bright at bookwork. *Headaches* also if constipated or having to hold urine for a long time in school. Tendency to make mistakes in writing, to transpose words or letters.

*Unreasoning* hatred of other child – no cause.

Better from *physical exertion*.

Poor at standing – faint, headachy or tired.

*Hunger* between meals causes headache; hunger in middle of night. In spite of eating they remain thin, small and fine.

Desire for *highly seasoned* food.

*Teeth* poor enamel, decay, abscesses.

Digestive upsets and diarrhoea, worse from *hot drinks*.

Irritant diarrhoea – sore anus and fissures.

*Rheumatic* complaints, worse from heat, better from motion. Numbness of limbs.

(Pulsatilla is heavier, softer, tired from exertion, chilled by cold water.)

**Arsenicum (Group 5)**

Highly strung, nervy, finely built, delicate looking with fine skin and hair.

Chilly, like to be covered but want head cool, especially with congestive headaches.

Scared, *frightened* of anything unusual, of the dark, being alone, going out alone. *Vivid* imagination. Night terrors.

Want to be comforted, consoled, somebody there.

*Restless.* Always doing something, going from one thing to another, or if nervous from one person to another.

Suddenly exhausted after activity, pale, wants to lie down, feels ill and frightened.

*Tidy* – hate mess – distressed out of all proportion.

Liable to catch cold.

Acute coryza, burning watery discharge, sneezing, tending to go rapidly into bronchitis, often with hoarseness between the cold and the chest symptoms.

*Or*, sudden acute tight *asthma* – terrified. Occurring 1–3 p.m. or a.m. Then frothy white sputum.

Very sensitive to cold which leads to respiratory or gastric symptoms.

Digestive upset from exposure to cold or following icecream and fruit.

Pains are eased by warmth, and they prefer warm drinks.

*Acute diarrhoea* may develop – sudden onset with collapse, restlessness, exhaustion after each frequent small stool, grey, cold and sweaty. In acute states a baby may only be able to move his head constantly back and forth.

*Hyperaesthesia* – sensitive to smell, touch, to noise, to excitement.

They will get sick, nervy or have nightmares.

If pushed at school, headaches periodical every 7 or 14 days, lasting a day or two and completely prostrated; intense congestive headache worse from noise, light or disturbance and, as already stated, better from cold air or cold cloth.


**Chamomilla (Group 5)**

The Chamomilla child has certain similarities to the Arsenicum child, but some characteristic differences.

*Hyperaesthesia*, acute sensitivity to *noise, pain* and people; intense pain which puts them into a frenzy of rage – they resent it, demand to have it removed and will strike you.

Intense *restlessness*, wants to be carried about, passed from one person to another, jogged up and down. Yells if you stop and pulls your hair. Never satisfied with anything he is doing, gets tired of it, throws it down.

More irritable and excitable about 9 p.m.

*Flushed*, when angry, with hot head and often *one cheek red*.

*Teething*, one of the great remedies for this; cross at night, tender inflamed gums, flush of one cheek, worse from hot application or hot room, better from *cold* application.

*Acute colic* – usually from anger, or after screaming; with wind and diarrhoea, green stools. Colic relieved by *hot* application (opposite for teething).

*Hot* children, hot head, hot burning feet which they stick out of bed.

May scream till they go blue or even have convulsions.

*Otitis* media: doesn't want to be touched, *very irritable*, yells with pain, again one-sided flush of face.

**Cina** (Vegetable, with Santonin as its principal substance) **(Group 5)**

| | Compare **Chamomilla** |
|---|---|
| Obstinacy | Unstable. |
| Circumscribed red patch on cheeks and pallor around mouth. | One red cheek. |
| Dislike of being handled or interference – *tender to touch*. | Mental resentment. |
| Steady passive motion soothes. | |
| *Sickness* but immediately after hungry. | |
| Nightmares and terrors if a late meal. | |
| *Diarrhoea* – white watery stool – particularly white. | Green stool. |
| Relief from pressure – lies on tummy with colic. | |

*Chilly* – sensitive to draughts.

Irregular twitching of face muscles after excitement.

Touchy – can't see a joke. (Older child.)

Hyperaesthesia of head and scalp – do *not* stroke. Jar aggravates.

*Yawning*. Acidosis.

Restless with digestive upset; meningeal irritation – rubbing head into pillow – may develop squint.

*Irritation* of nose – red, itchy, picking it (not necessarily worms).

**Magnesia Carbonica (Group 5)**

Sensitive, nervous type of child with lack of stamina, poor muscular power and soft flabby muscles. Any physical exertion tires them out. Easily startled by unexpected touch. Sensitive to the cold, but better in the open air, and upset by changes in the weather. Flush and sweat of the face after hot food or drink.

Headaches. Violent, neuralgic, pains tending to come on at night, with marked *sleeplessness*. The older child is mentally tired out at school.

Adolescents are dead beat in the morning and difficult to get to school.
Desire for meat or meaty tastes.
Aversion to vegetables.
Intolerance to milk; sour vomiting and pale, pasty undigested stools, *white* soft and like putty or eventually watery and excoriating. (Cina has white stools also.)
Tendency to *bronchitis* with enteritis – stringy, difficult sputum like Kali Bich.
Skin *dry*, scaly, copper-coloured eruption of the scalp.

### Ignatia (Group 5)

This remedy is often thought of only for hysterical women, but it has a much wider application, and can be useful in children who are highly strung, bright, sensitive and precocious. They do well at school, but if pushed they start to react with nervous headaches. The headache comes on later in the day and is relieved by heat.

Although clever, they blame themselves if they start to go to pieces, and become depressed and melancholy. In a confined place, they get nervous, distressed, choky and faint. Strained expression, tendency to grimace, twitch of eyelid or blinking.

Writing may become shaky when under stress. Up in the air or down in the dumps. Very *sensitive* to noise, cannot stand this while studying, blows up and then weepy, and then quite unable to concentrate or think. Scared if they get nervous – afraid of something going to happen, of taking initiative or going out alone.

*Digestive* upsets – sometimes upset by simplest foods and yet eats and digests most indigestible food. (Contradictions.)
Also inflamed throat, relieved by solid food pressing on it.
*Cough*, irritating, spasmodic – on and on, or acute laryngitis.
Rheumatic pains, better from firm pressure.

### Zincum (Group 5)

A nervous, sensitive, excitable kind of child. The Ignatia child is very bright and quick, the Zinc child is slow in reacting, slow in grasping what you are saying, slow in answering, more docile and less unstable than Ignatia. Delayed development, especially delayed puberty.

*Tired* physically and mentally. When tired they get a persistent aching pain in the lower cervical region, with burning pain down the back.
*Cramp* in the hamstring muscles in bed.
*Restless, twitchy, fidgety* – restless feet.
*Chilly*, very sensitive to cold.

Inflamed eyes from the cold, with chronic blepharitis, and intense photophobia.

Sensitive to *noise* especially *talking*. When the child is working talking drives them distracted.

Generalised skin eruption in childhood followed by chorea in adolescence.

Acute hunger at 11 a.m.

Tendency to bolt their food.

# Chapter 21

# *The Nosodes*

## THE BOWEL NOSODES

These remedies were developed originally by Edward Bach and then by Dr John Paterson of Glasgow, a bacteriologist as well as a physician. He was assisted in this work by his wife Elizabeth, and both published papers in the *British Homoeopathic Journal*.

The remedies were originally derived from cultures of stools, and were prescribed on the basis of the percentages of organisms found in the stools of patients. Since the advent of antibiotics it has been found difficult to grow non-lactose fermenting organisms from stools, so the remedies are now used mainly on certain clinical indications, or on their association with related remedies. It is usually recommended that a single dose should be given and not repeated for several months, using related remedies in the interval. They can also be used as a starting remedy, where the picture of symptoms is not sufficiently clear to select a single remedy, but where the nosode covers a likely group of remedies, e.g. Morgan Co. (or Compound).

The bowel nosodes are usually prescribed in 30c potency.

### Bacillus No. 7
*Mental and physical fatigue.*
Unfit for mental effort leading to extreme physical exhaustion.
Flatulence, fullness after food.
Feeble urinary flow, loss of sexual function, premature senility.
Asthma, catarrh, sticky mucus.
Low BP and myocardial weakness.
Rheumatic nodules, backache, cannot stand long, faints easily. Sensitive to cold.
Related remedies are, Bromine, Iodine and particularly the Kali salts, especially Kali Carb.

### Dysentery Co.
The keynote of this remedy is *nervous tension*, particularly anticipatory in character. The patient has a tense facial expression, not fearful but

alert and ready to react. He is anxious, restless, fidgety, timid and uneasy amongst strangers; easily upset by criticism. Involuntary movements, tics or twitchings (like chorea) occur. There is instability of the capillary circulation, causing blushing, frontal headaches from excitement and claustrophobia. The skin may be dry, scaly and with circinate lesions.

Its most marked sphere of action is in pyloric spasm, and where pyloric stenosis is spasmodic rather than mechanical (where surgical operation is often required). There is dilatation of the stomach, vomiting and a 1 a.m. aggravation time. Often valuable in duodenal ulcer, particularly when the pain and spasm follow anticipatory or nervous tension. In adults cardiac disorders with mental tension and palpitation may be helped.

We see the close relationship between Dysentery Co. and Argentum Nit. and Arsenicum Alb. It is also related to Kalmia. Nux Vomica and Lycopodium also follow it well in gastric disorders.

## Gaertner (Bach)

This remedy is very valuable in malnutrition, either from lack of adequate diet or failure to metabolise, e.g. in steatorrhoea, coeliac disease or following gastric operations, and in some cases of colitis. Correction of diet, and vitamin and protein supplements are essential, but Gaertner helps the assimilation of these. It used to be of value in marasmic children, and may well have a place in underdeveloped countries and among refugees with inadequate diet. Emaciation in malignant disease and in the elderly is a further indication.

The children are hypersensitive to all impressions, physical and psychical, with fear of the dark and being alone. They have active brains, although poorly nourished bodies and poor muscular development. They are restless – wandering about looking at things, but their attention is not held.

The remedies most closely associated with this nosode are Phosphorus, Silica and Mercurius.

## Morgan Co. (Bach)

The keynote of this remedy is *congestion*. It is selective on skin and liver, in headaches with flushed face, aggravation from heat and raised blood pressure. The congestive features are seen in bronchopneumonia, where the indicated remedy fails to act even in the acute state, or to clear up a residual infection; and in pelvic congestion and dysmenorrhoea, flushes of the menopause, circulatory disturbances of the limbs, blueness, chilblains, varicose veins, oedema and hot feet, etc., skin ailments with heat and itch – eczema, red, raw with exudate, itching and bleeding. Hence the relationship to Sulphur with its hyperaemia of the surface circulation, Carbon with its deep internal venous stasis, Graphites, Petroleum and Psorinum.

In the digestive sphere: congestion of the stomach lining and the liver with dirty mouth, indigestion and bilious vomiting. A great remedy in gallbladder conditions, constipation and piles.

These patients have a red coarse blotchy appearance, are often introspective, anxious about their health and irritable with a tendency to depression.

It can be helpful in the congestion around the joints in arthritis. There are two sub-types of this nosode – Morgan Pure, which is closest to Sulphur and particularly good in skin conditions, and Morgan Gaertner, which is like Lycopodium and is helpful in cholecystitis and renal colic. It is often useful in hiatus hernia and diverticular disease.

Sometimes giving the nosode Morgan Co. in 30c potency, followed by Sulphur in 3x or 6x tablets twice daily, can help the acute itching in bad eczema or dermatitis.

**Proteus**
The keynote of this remedy is *suddenness* and *violence*, with nervous symptoms and spasm.

Violent temper in a child with kicking. Emotional hysteria such as one connects with Ignatia and Natrum Mur., and petit mal attacks of epilepsy.

The element of spasm in peripheral vessels makes it valuable in Raynaud's Syndrome, along with Secale, and in some cases of cramp. Migrainous headaches with blurred vision and Menière's syndrome may be helped.

In the skin we find herpetic eruptions with pain out of proportion to the lesion, and angioneurotic oedema.

In the digestive sphere the sudden onset is important, either haemorrhage or perforation, without any previous stomach symptoms but with a history of nervous strain building up. This slow build up of strain in business and society with a sudden catastrophe is typical of Western countries today. Needless to say the patient with severe haemorrhage or perforation may require transfusion or surgical intervention.

Related remedies are Ignatia, Natrum Mur., Apis, Cuprum.

**Sycotic Co.** (from non-lactose fermenting cocci of intestinal tract)
The keynote here is 'irritation', particularly in relation to mucous membranes. Hence its value in all catarrhal states of the respiratory tract, the bladder and the vagina, asthma, sinusitis, enuresis, chronic cystitis, vulvovaginitis, leucorrhoea, albuminuria, gastroenteritis. We also find it of value in warty growths, enlarged lymphoid tissue of tonsils and adenoids, glands, and the irritation of synovial linings in rheumatism; meningeal irritation, convulsions.

The patients are pale, sallow, flabby and soft, with long eyelashes (like Tuberculinum Bov.) and sweat of the head.

Stools are excoriating, loose and offensive, with urgent call to stool on rising.

Cough occurs about 2 a.m. and is worse from change of atmosphere, and symptoms generally are worse from damp.

There is fear, irritability and temper.

The related sycotic remedies are Thuja, Nitric Acid, Natrum Sulph. and Bacillinum.


## NOSODES FROM DISEASED TISSUE

These are remedies prepared from diseased tissue or infected discharges. They are potentised and do not contain active organisms, and are therefore quite safe. There are two main groups. The first are used either in prophylaxis or, more commonly, as a follow-up to an acute infectious illness, having no real symptom picture or proving. The other group have a distinct symptomalogy on which to prescribe.

**Group I**
>    Morbillinum – related to measles.
>    Diphtherinum – related to diphtheria.
>    Scarlatinum – related to scarlet fever.
>    Parotidinum – related to mumps.
>    Pertussin – related to whooping cough.
>    Variolinum – related to smallpox.
>    Influenzinum – related to influenza.

Recently added are:

>    Rubella nosode.
>    Glandular fever nosode.
>    Brucella abortus nosode.

Also:

>    Staphylococcin.
>    Stretococcin.
>    E. coli nosode.

These are all used where a patient has *never been well since* a particular infection or has persistent sepsis. They are not generally used during the acute illness, when the indicated remedy should be given.

Potencies of allergens are now available and are used in single occasional doses where indicated. For example: house dust or dust mite, pollens, grasses, dog hair, cat fur, horse hair, moulds.

Remedies potentised from drugs or metals may be used to antidote the side effects or allergic reactions of specific substances. For example:

Penicillium.
Cortisone.
Soap powder and detergents.
Nickel.

## Group II

This group contains nosodes which have a fuller drug picture, and which may be used either on the symptom picture or if there is a past or family history of that illness.

Tuberculinum or Bacillinum.
Medorrhinum (gonorrhoeal nosode).
Syphilinum (Lueticum).
Psorinum.
Carcinosin.

Most of these are described in more detail in Section III.

# SECTION III

# MATERIA MEDICA

This section contains the symptom pictures of some of the leading homoeopathic remedies. These are only summaries, and in order to learn the full picture of the remedy, and in particular its 'essence', it is necessary to study the remedy in several texts. The most useful are:

*Introduction to the Principles and Practice of Homoeopathy* C. E. Wheeler and J. D. Kenyon.
*Homoeopathic Drug Pictures*    Margaret Tyler.
*Leaders in Homoeopathic Therapeutics*    E. B. Nash.
*The Patient not the Cure*    Margery Blackie.
*Lectures on Homoeopathic Materia Medica*    J. T. Kent.

These texts describe each remedy in the totality of symptoms. They also explain the principal mental and emotional states and types of individuals who most benefit from that particular remedy. This is the 'essence' of the remedy, the grasp of which is so vital in chronic prescribing.

# Chapter 22

# *Fifty Common Remedies Described in Greater Detail*

## ALUMINA

This remedy is one of the great antipsorics, like Graphites and Sulphur. It is an antidote to lead.

Although experiments to assess the amount of aluminium absorbed by cooking in aluminium pans suggest that there is only a slight increase over the normal physiological levels, there do seem to be people who are sensitive to it, and who are made ill by eating food cooked in aluminium utensils.

Characteristically the Alumina patient has a pale, greyish metallic look, often dry, wrinkled and old looking.

DRYNESS runs through its symptoms, in the skin, the respiratory and digestive tracts.

It is a remedy of paresis, ptosis of the eyelids (Causticum), intestinal paralysis (Plumbum), causing slowness in passing urine, constipation and weakness, mental and physical, with heaviness of the legs.

A chilly remedy, but with a liking for open air.

### Mentals
The mental symptoms described vary from one text to another. They are intellectual, but with dulled intellect in the morning, and alert by the evening, when they become more fearful and apprehensive.

Kent describes a confused dazed state with a feeling of unreality (Medorrhinum), unable to make decisions, sad, yet they may be hurried, with impulses to kill on seeing a knife.

Hypochondriacal men with lassitude and indifference to work, peevish.

### Eyes
The eyelids are inflamed, sticky, burning, dry, with the lashes falling out.

### Respiratory
There is dryness of the mucous membranes of the nose and throat, with a stuffed up nose, and headache from chronic catarrh, the headache

often on the vertex, better from pressure, and accompanied
sometimes by vertigo.

Dry hacking cough worse in the morning, with hoarseness especially in
singers. (Argentum Met. has a similar hacking cough and hoarseness
during the day.)

## Gastrointestinal

A feeling of constriction in the lower oesophagus.

Loss of appetite, eructations, eats indigestible things.

Desires – fruit and vegetables.

Aversion – meat.

Aggravation from potatoes and irritating things like salt, vinegar,
pepper, spirits and tobacco.

*Constipation* – No desire, no power to strain even with a soft stool –
excoriation of anus with soft stool.

## Skin

The skin is rough and dry with eruptions which crack, itch and burn and
are worse from the warmth of the bed.

## APIS (From the Sting of the Honey Bee)

This remedy mainly affects the skin and serous membranes, throat, kidneys, meninges, pericardium and joints.

It is characterised by BURNING, STINGING pains, with redness and marked swelling and OEDEMA. There is great SENSITIVITY to touch in all areas except the head (which is relieved by pressure), and there is general soreness leading to RESTLESSNESS (like Rhus Tox., but not relieved by motion).

HEAT in any form AGGRAVATES; hot room, hot bath, hot applications. Violent sudden onset.

### Mentals
Conditions resulting from grief, fright, anger, jealousy, suppressed eruptions.

Tearful, depressed, anxious, constant weeping and whining.

May be irritable, suspicious, jealous.

As infections become more severe the patient is listless, apathetic, indifferent and eventually stuporose.

In meningitis there is muttering delirium with sudden piercing cries. All the mental symptoms are made worse by heat.

### Head
Hot and congested with sudden, stabbing pains worse on movement and better from pressure (other symptoms worse from touch).

### Eyes
Inflammatory conditions of eyes, iritis, keratitis, trachoma, with redness, oedema of lids, burning stinging pains relieved by cold.

### Face
Red, burning and stinging; of value in erysipelas.

In kidney disease the face is pale and waxy.

### Tongue
Fiery hot red or dry and trembling.

### Throat
Red, smooth swelling with oedematous uvula, burning stinging pain, again worse from heat and better from cold.

*Absence of thirst* even in fever.

### Respiratory
Violent dry spasmodic cough with soreness and sensitivity of the larynx. Sensation of suffocation.

**Genito-urinary**

Nephritis with marked oedema, with restlessness, drowsiness and lack of thirst.

Neuralgia of ovaries especially right; dysmenorrhoea.

**Skin**

Urticaria. Itching intolerable, swelling marked, stinging burning pain and sensitivity to touch.

**Limbs**

Trembling, twitching and jerking of muscle groups.

Inflammation of synovial membranes of joints, swollen, shiny; sharp stinging pains, sensitivity and marked effusion. Restless, worse from heat.

## ARGENTUM NITRICUM

### Generals
HEAT aggravates – hates stuffy place.
Desires cold air, cold drinks, cold food.

### Mentals
A remedy with many nervous symptoms, particularly the excitement of anticipation of events, causing diarrhoea.

Irrational, does strange things, or foolish things; troublesome thoughts which make him hurry – walks faster and faster.

Fear of death, of crowded enclosed places, church, high places. Feels he might jump down. Feels high buildings will fall on him.

Overworked, overtired, mental exhaustion and trembling.

### Head
Brain fag and headache worse from heat, but likes head tightly bound.

### Gastrointestinal
Desires *sweet*, especially sugar, which causes diarrhoea, and salt, strong tasting foods.

Flatulence and distension marked.

Pains in abdomen, epigastric and spreading to the left.

Worse after eating, better from vomiting.

Vomiting and diarrhoea together (like Arsenicum Alb.).

Diarrhoea often greenish, like chopped spinach.

Tongue either smooth, red and sore, or pale, dry and flabby.

Ulcerations; mucous membranes, mouth, bladder, stomach with bleeding.

### Other symptoms
*Eyes* often affected; ulceration, purulent discharge.

Worse from heat, better from cold.

Sensation of stick in the throat (like Hepar Sul.) but relieved by cold.

Palpitation lying on the right side.

Worse before and during menses with dysmenorrhoea from excitement, and heavy bleeding.

Numbness of the arms at night – also hyperaesthesia.

## ARNICA MONTANA

This remedy is mainly known for its action in injury and bruising, but it has wider indications.

It is a remedy to be thought of in any form of trauma, after surgical operations, following the trauma of a cerebral haemorrhage or a myocardial infarction, in rheumatism, gout and in the elderly.

### Mentals
Irritable, morose, sad, does not want to be touched.

Forgetfulness, absentmindedness, hopelessness, indifference. Sudden horror of instant death – in cardiac disease. Dreadful dreams and imaginings – will relive the horrors of an accident.

*Says he feels well* – when seriously ill.

Cold nose.

Head burning hot with a cold body.

Great fear of *being touched* because of sensitiveness, e.g. gout.

### Head
Cerebral haemorrhage – before it, pain as if the head was distended from within.

Haemorrhages in the eye; easy bleeding; ecchymoses.

### Respiratory
Whooping cough – painful cough, spasmodic with blood-stained sputum, bruised feeling with aggravation from touch. Child is cross and fretful.

Stitching pains in the chest like Bryonia, but worse from touch.

### Gastrointestinal
Foul breath and taste in typhoid-like illnesses, with stupor and coma.

Offensive flatus and stool and eructations.

### Other symptoms
*Restlessness* because the *bed feels hard*. The soreness is relieved by change of position. (Rhus Tox. must move – uneasiness better from moving. Arsenicum Alb. anxious, no relief even when moving.)

Sensation as if bruised or beaten all over.

General weakness and weariness – of value in the elderly.

Pains in the limbs and joints in rheumatism, sore as if bruised.

Effects of overfatigue, physical or mental.

Can be applied locally for wasp sting – better in lc potency diluted 5–10 drops in a pint of water. Too long application may cause dermatitis.

## ARSENICUM ALBUM

These patients are always extremely fastidious in their appearance, dress and habits. This is noticeable in their house or garden.

RESTLESSNESS, BURNING, PROSTRATION, MIDNIGHT AGGRAVATION.

Extreme *chilliness*, cold hands, rigors and chills like ice water going through him, with thirst during the sweat, but not much during the heat.

Cold air aggravates, except for the head which prefers air.

*Restlessness* is a constant symptom, hurried, pours out his story.

Prostration *out of all proportion* when symptoms appear trivial.

*Burnings* in all parts, better from heat. Discharges are acrid and corrosive – nose, eyes, leucorrhoea, from ulcers.

Aggravation *midnight* and *1 a.m.*

### Mentals
*Anguish*. Anxiety for himself – feels it is useless to take medicine, as he is sure to die.

Sensitive to smells, touch, surroundings – fastidious in habits, dress. Hair is soft and beautifully kept.

### Respiratory
Asthma; must sit up, breathless on moving, sharp pain in the right upper lung.

Suffocative catarrh on lying down.

### Gastric
Vomiting and diarrhoea, acute stomach and bowel pains, food poisoning. Thirst for small drinks, especially *warm*.

### Other symptoms
Bleedings anywhere.

Oedema with thirst (Apis without thirst).

May help pain and restlessness in inoperable cancers.

May bring back old suppressed eruptions (e.g. eczema).

## AURUM METALLICUM

The main characteristic of all Aurum salts is suicidal depression with want of self-confidence, alternating with hysteria and a kind of hysterical excitement and anger. They are restless and hurried mentally, but aggravated from physical hurry.

Desire for open air (except Aurum Sulph.). Better from cold and cool applications, yet icy cold hands and feet. Aggravation on waking (like Lachesis).

### Mentals
Irritable and in particular angry at contradiction.

Full of self-condemnation, but extremely critical of others.

The hysteria or depression may be brought on by anxiety, fear or contradiction.

Sulky, indisposed to talk, sits apart, weeping, meditates on death.

Discontented with circumstances, quarrelsome.

Apprehensive fear, hypersensitive to noise, which makes her anxious, dread of men.

Terrifying dreams of death, thieves, falling from a height.

### Eyes
Ulceration of cornea, and inflammation of iris.

### Ears
Noises in ears.

### Respiratory
Catarrhs; ulceration of nose and offensive discharge, everything smells too strong – has a putrid smell from his own nose. Nose red and swollen. Metallic taste.

### Stomach
Craving for alcohol and feels better for it (useful in alcoholics).

### Skin
Deep ulceration of skin, and malignant skin lesions.

Induration of glands.

### Rheumatic
Deep boring, tearing pains in bones and rheumatic joints, worse at night.

### Other symptoms
Serious heart conditions and chronic nephritis, with albumen and blood in urine. Sterility.

The Aurum state may come on after syphilis, and from loss of property or fear of this.

Note the many similar symptoms to those in Syphilinum.

## BARYTA CARBONICA

A remedy of children and old age.

CHILLINESS, sensitive to cold except PRESSING HEADACHE which is better in the open air.

Emaciation, weakness. Pale, withered face.

ENLARGED GLANDS particularly tonsillar but also generalised, chronic and indurated. Also mesenteric.

Degenerative conditions, cardiovascular, aneurysm, cerebral.

Prostatic hypertrophy.

**Mentals**

In child, slow learning to walk.

Slowness of maturing in adolescent and young adult.

Mental dwarfishness.

Loss of memory, mental weakness, confusion, loss of confidence. Aversion to strangers, shy child, timid.

Premature old age – childlike behaviour in old.

Want of clear consciousness in elderly – not clear in his intellect.

The *child* hides, easily frightened, imagines all sorts of strange things, cannot comprehend or memorise.

Sits and sits, lack of ability to think. Fear of something going to happen (Causticum). Whining, hatching up complaints and grievances.

*Thinking of troubles* makes them worse.

**Ears**

Noises, crackling when swallowing, associated with enlarged tonsils and glands.

**Mouth and throat**

Dry mouth, bad taste, burning tongue. Weakness and paralysis of tongue in old people.

*Throat:* Chronic suppuration, slow onset, granular looking.

Blocking and gagging with solid food.

Spasm in the oesophagus when food goes down – in the elderly.

**Respiratory**

Coryza with swollen upper lips, thick yellow mucus, scabs and bleeding.

Weakness of voice, huskiness.

Dry suffocative cough. *Rattling in trachea* aggravated by cold weather.

Cannot expectorate. (Senega, Ammoniacum, Baryta Mur.)

**Heart**

Palpitation worse lying on the left side, and worse thinking of it.

**Gastrointestinal**
Weakness of digestion, distension, wind, hiccup and pain after food.
*Constipation:* Lack of action, knotty stools, piles protrude.

**Other symptoms**
Granular, sticky eyelids.
Dry eruption on the scalp in infants.
Gouty rheumatic pains, worse from cold.
Offensive perspiration of feet, causing soreness, ulceration.

## BRYONIA

There are certain marked characteristics of this remedy. Intense AGGRAVATION from any MOVEMENT. This applies to headache, to joint pains, to pleurisy and, in the mental sphere, to any disturbance or exertion.

DRYNESS of serous or mucous membranes – dry mouth, dry intestinal mucosa with hard stools, dry cough and dry pleurisy. COLD, DRY, east WINDS aggravate and yet most Bryonia symptoms are worse in warm weather, warm room or getting overheated. There is a general relief from cold, cold applications.

PRESSURE relieves – joint, headache, chest pain, except abdominal pains which are worse from pressure.

Time aggravation at 9 p.m. or early morning, 3 a.m.

### Mentals
Bad temper and irritability, dislikes being disturbed when acutely ill, will not talk if he can help it. When seriously ill with pneumonia or fever he will be still like a log, with dulled senses and intellect, and resenting any interference or questioning. Fits of anger, weak memory, delirium and dreams of his business or events of the day. A child keeps wanting something and does not know what. Despondent, anxious with fear of death and despair of recovery.

### Headache
Severe dull throbbing pain, with acute stabs over the eyes, relieved by hard pressure and cool applications, worse from movement and any exertion of mind or body.

### Fever
Of value in influenza, pneumonia, typhoid and typhus. Marked *thirst* for large quantities at long intervals, profuse sour perspiration, dry lips and mouth with white or yellow tongue, and delirium and mental symptoms described above.

### Respiratory
Laryngitis and tracheitis with hoarseness and dry cough which is worse on entering a warm room and better from cool air. (Opposite of Phosphorus.)

Pleurisy with sharp, stitching pains in the chest, better from pressure or lying on the affected side (which prevents movement).

In pneumonia the patient looks heavy and dusky, with dry mouth, white tongue, thirst and perspiration and always better from cold air and cold applications.

**Gastrointestinal**

Pain and discomfort in the liver region, and even jaundice, epigastric pain and in this instance worse from pressure.

Nausea, waterbrash and sour eructations, dirty yellow tongue and thirst for cold, although the stomach symptoms are really more relieved by warm fluid.

Stools dry and crumbling.

All alimentary symptoms are again worse from movement.

**Rheumatism**

Muscles, fibrous tissue and joint synovium affected, with pain, redness, heat and swelling from effusion, and all aggravated by movement.

Pain is worse from moving. (Opposite of Rhus Tox.).

In acute rheumatism there is sour perspiration, and irritability. Sometimes local heat will help but more often cold applications relieve the pain.

Bryonia is often the acute of Natrum Mur., and is followed well by Natrum Mur. after the acute phase is over (e.g. in migraine).

### CALCAREA CARBONICA (Impure Calcium Carbonate from the middle layer of the oyster shell)

Calcarea patients are always susceptible to COLD, and dread the open air. The least cold, and especially COLD DAMP weather, aggravates their symptoms. Cold clammy feet, although they can burn when warm at night. Hands are soft, moist, 'boneless' feeling and cold; chilblains frequent. There is SLOWNESS, mentally and bodily, in movement, thought, learning and growth. Physical and mental exertion exhausts.

Tendency to catch cold easily, to develop enlarged glands, polypi, leg ulcers and varicose veins.

Aggravation at 2–3 a.m.

The INFANT is fat, flabby and pale with a big head, slow closure of the fontanelles, and delayed dentition. Crusty eruption on the scalp. Chilliness with profuse perspiration of the head, soaking the pillow. Cough in teething children. Night terrors, sees things and wakes up screaming.

The ADULT Calcarea is also pale, flabby, phlegmatic, not necessarily fat but with a big head and scraggy neck.

Breathless, anaemic, chilly with tendency to palpitation.

## Mentals

The child is lethargic, dull and just sits. She is clumsy, easily scared, sensitive to criticism or being laughed at and feels useless. Also the night terrors mentioned.

Older people are depressed, sluggish mentally, full of fears; that she will lose her reason, of getting a cerebral haemorrhage, of what will happen, of the dark. Worries over others, over silly things, sensitive to injustice done to others. Tears trickle silently down the face. Peevish, obstinate, cannot think or remember – pauses before replying. May give up work, lean back and let others look after them – parents may do this with their daughter, although really quite able to do things for themselves.

## Head

Vertigo and faint feelings. Headaches.

## Eyes

Photophobia, sore in a cold wind; cataract.

## Respiratory

Chronic catarrh, nasal polypi, enlarged tonsils and adenoids.

Dry, irritating cough with pains in the larynx and chest, worse at night with wheezing and gasping.

**Gastrointestinal**

Desire for eggs. Eats indigestible things like chalk, coal and earth (children). Later in life they dislike meat, coffee and milk. Milk disagrees. They must have a good breakfast or they get headaches.

*Sour* vomit, sour taste, dry white coated tongue.

Distended abdomen. Constipation but always feels better when constipated (laxatives upset).

Sour smelling excoriating diarrhoea.

**Genitals**

Profuse and early menses.

Thick acrid leucorrhoea.

**Limbs**

Trembling, twitching, spasms. *Cramps* in the feet and calves on walking or in bed.

Weak ankles, pains in the long bones, wrists and between the scapulae. Back feels as if beaten.

Belladonna is the acute of Calcarea Carbonica and would be used in an acute illness, and followed up by Calcarea. Calcarea Carb. is also a chronic remedy related to Rhus Tox.

## CALCAREA PHOSPHORICA

One of Schuessler's tissue salts, containing lime and phosphorus, and an essential for nutrition, growth and healing of bones.

In a small child there is slowness to develop and learn, slowness in closing of fontanelles, sunken abdomen, weakness of the neck and limbs and sweating. Colic in INFANTS after eating and watery, green slimy hot, spluttering stools.

THE OLDER CHILD is thin, dark, but may be fair with blue eyes, growing with long legs, pains in the limbs. Cold limbs and face. Clammy skin, greasy (like suet pudding). The rheumatic pains are worse from cold, moving, in spring and autumn – with aching numbness and cramps. Neuralgic face pains better from heat, but worse on exertion and pressure. Muscular growing pains.

**Mentals**
The child is restless, going back and forth, reluctant to talk, tired with weak memory, discontented, peevish – always complaining that something is wrong (with school, etc.). Full of vague fears and dreads – especially in the evening. Indisposition to work, cannot concentrate. Anxiety causes tummy upset and diarrhoea.

**Headaches**
In schoolgirls aggravated by mental effort, exposure to draughts, cold air, feeling of ice in the back of the neck. Amelioration of headache from bathing in cold water, worse from pressure, jar, exertion, tight hat.

**Respiratory**
Tickly cough – sputum yellow, offensive, worse in cold weather; head sweats, bronchospasm, better from lying down, worse on getting up. Pedunculated polyps. Glands in the neck. Chronic catarrh, better in a warm room, worse from cold.

**Stomach**
Good appetite. Desires tasty food, ham rind, kippers (not so much salt as Phosphorus).
Upset by ice-cream, cold drinks.

**Menses**
Slow maturing and painful menstruation (cramping better with the flow).

## CARBO VEGETABILIS (Wood Charcoal, inert until triturated)

Hahnemann used only a 3c potency. Carbo Veg. affects mainly the vascular system, especially the venous circulation. Everything about the patient is SLUGGISH, lazy, full, distended, swollen and puffed. The hands are puffed, the veins are full, the body feels full and turgid, the head feels full, the limbs feel full so that the patient wants to put his feet up. There are varicose veins and ulceration with blackish or bluish patches, stagnation in the veins, poor tissues.

### Generals
*Burnings* internally, in veins, head, skin, inflamed parts, stomach.
But *icy coldness* of the nose, tongue, breath, knees and feet.
Collapse with cold sweat, cold face and breath.
Vital force nearly exhausted.
Blueness of the face.

### Mentals
The mental state is slow, sluggish, stupid, lazy.
Great indifference.

### Head
Headaches mainly occipital, feeling of a weight, dislikes the pressure of a hat.

### Respiratory
Dyspnoea with expectoration, exhausting sweating and great coldness.
Acute violent spasmodic cough in paroxysms with cold sweat and cold pinched face.
Very useful in *whooping cough.*
In acute asthma and cardiac failure the patient wants to sit at the window or be *fanned*, even although he is cold and sweaty.

### Gastrointestinal
One of the great *flatulent* remedies, full, distended with belching of wind, worse at night.
Acid risings in the night. Offensive flatus. (Carbo Animalis is often better for relieving the flatulence after surgical operations.)
Desire for coffee, acid foods, sweet, salt.
Loves to eat indigestible foods like puddings, pies, sauce and is averse to digestible food.
Offensive green diarrhoea.

A most valuable remedy for a collapsed patient, in a faint or even a heart attack, or post-operatively, where he is cold, pale, sweaty with a thready pulse, but wanting air.

CAUSTICUM (Potash preparation. See Hahnemann's instructions in Tyler.)

Sallow, sickly-looking, dark hair, dark eyes, dark mood. Paralysis, contractures, rheumatoid, warts.
After suppression of eruptions. Broken-down constitution.

## Generals
*Worse in cold dry winds*, frost, causing paralysis, rheumatism.

## Mentals
Hopeless, weepy, foreboding, apprehension, despair of recovery, fear something going to happen, fear of dark, twilight.
Irritable, peevish and distrustful, but very sympathetic to suffering of others.
Ailments from grief, loss of sleep, anger. May sit silently, inattentive.
Memory fails and mental effort leads to symptoms.

## Vertigo
Worse on lying down in bed, worse on stooping, worse at menses: tendency to fall forwards or sideways. Sensation of space between brain and skull, better from warmth.

## Paralysis
Of single parts – *facial*, swallowing, voice – throat, eyelids, limbs with trembling. (All like Gelsemium.) Especially after exposure to very cold wind.

## Eyes
Dry, stinging, itching, wants to dab eyelids.

## Respiratory
Hoarseness worse in the morning (Phosphorus evening). Burning rawness. Loss of voice. Inability to raise sputum, partly raised and slips back. Urine spurts on coughing. Cough relieved by cold water.

## Stomach
Sits down hungry but smell of food upsets (Arsenicum, Sepia, Cocculus).

## Rectum
Paralysis – inactive, fills up, no desire – better standing up.

**Genito-urinary**

A most valuable remedy in cystitis – acute sensitiveness to cold. Great urgency with inability to pass urine, then later on involuntary passage of urine without warning. Shooting pain in rectum when cannot pass urine.

Incontinence on coughing, sneezing or exertion.

Valuable following operation, when patient cannot pass urine.

Menstrual colic with tearing back pains better at night. Epilepsy with incontinence during irregular menses.

**Warts**

Hands, face, nose, eyes, large, bleed easily. (Thuja, Dulcamara.)

**Rheumatic**

Advanced with contractures of tendons, drawing pains, cannot get ease, restless at night. Worse in dry cold. Better from warmth and wet.

## CHELIDONIUM MAJUS (Greater Celandine)

This remedy is best known for its effects in cases of jaundice or liver trouble and as a pneumonia remedy.

The most characteristic symptom is a fixed pain, either dull or sharp, under the lower inner angle of the right scapula. This may occur in hepatitis or gallbladder disease or in cases of pneumonia.

### Headache
Mainly in the forehead and associated with biliousness or vomiting, brought on by heat and aggravated in a warm room or from warm applications.

### Respiratory
In many ways resembles Bryonia in pneumonia. Right basal inflammation, with stitching pleural pain, especially below the right scapula. The patient sits up perfectly still, as any movement causes pain, but unlike Bryonia, which likes pressure to the painful part, Chelidonium is worse from touch. Soon the patient will develop signs of jaundice or yellowness of the skin. Here there is relief from heat.

### Gastrointestinal
Bitter taste in the mouth. Tongue thickly coated, yellow with imprints of teeth round the edge. (Mercurius.) Tendency to jaundice, stools whitish in colour, tenderness or stitching pain in the liver and gallbladder area extending to the right scapula. It may relieve the pain in cholecystitis or gallstone colic.

Desire for hot drinks, hot milk or warm food.

### Other Symptoms
Rheumatic and neuralgic pains in the limbs.
Great weariness and drowsiness.

## CHINA (Cinchona Bark)

Chilly, sallow or jaundiced looking patient.
Pallor, weakness, nervous, sensitive to touch, motion, cold air; always catching colds, bowel and liver upsets.

### Debility
From loss of fluids, haemorrhage, sweating, diarrhoea, salivation, seminal emissions, purgatives. (not the weakness of anaemia – Ferrum; not the nervous debility of Phosphoric Acid; not the weakness from loss of sleep and nursing, which indicate Cocculus; not the strain of over-exertion or overwork of Arnica; but effects of loss of fluid.)

### Hyperaesthesia
Extreme pain sensitivity, aggravated by *touch* or moving but better from *firm pressure*, e.g. in headache or abdominal distension.

### Generals
Periodicity of symptoms – every other day.
Intermittent fevers – chill followed by fever, followed by sweat.
Thirst during the sweat, but not during the fever.
Persistent chilliness after influenza.

### Mentals
Emotional hyperaesthesia – dislike of company and a desire to be alone.
Timid disposition, imagines people are being critical when they look at him.
Considers himself ill-used, which leads to tempers, but not with the violence of Nux Vomica.

### Gastrointestinal
Tongue flabby and coated, yellowish white.
Diarrhoea; painless, undigested, profuse watery stools with marked debility.
Flatulent distension *not* relieved by flatus or eructation.

### Other symptoms
Haemorrhages, venous in type, menorrhagia, post-partum.
Ringing in the ears. (China or China Sulph. of value in Menière's syndrome.)

## CONIUM MACULATUM (Hemlock)

A deep acting remedy.
Paralysis, induration, glands. Hard infiltrated glands, breast lumps, induration of ulcers. Induration of testicles, impotency.

### Mentals
Weakness of memory, progressive, mind becomes tired, cannot concentrate or stand any mental effort.
Complete indifference.
Unhappiness. Slowly developing weakness of mind.
Will sit and mope in a corner.
Peevish, everything vexes him.
Any excitement brings on physical or mental distress.
Hysteria and hypochondriasis in widows or widowers denied sexual outlet.

### Vertigo
When turning head. Worse lying as though bed turned in a circle, worse on moving eyes, better when eyes closed.
Sick headache on watching moving objects, cars.

### Eyes
Weakness of eye muscles and lids, induration of lids.
*Photophobia* without inflammation – out of all proportion.

### Gastrointestinal
Paralysis of oesophagus – food stops on the way down; feeling of pressure rising from stomach in nervous women.
Constipation – ineffectual urging, hard stool, paralysis of rectum, cannot expel contents.

### Urinary
Urine flow will stop and start.

### Other symptoms
Cough dry, worse lying in bed.
*Numbness* with pains, or weakness. *Painless* complaints.
Weakness and increasing paralysis of muscles.
Stitching pains in head.
Tremblings, jerking and twitching.
Aching in legs from rheumatism or ulceration relieved by *letting legs hang down.*
Sweat *during* sleep – copious.

## CUPRUM METALLICUM

*Cramps, spasms, convulsions* (cholera, whooping cough), twitchings.
VIOLENCE OF SYMPTOMS.
All symptoms RELIEVED BY COLD DRINK, (whoop spasm).
Dyspnoea, bluish lips, icy cold; violent spasmodic cough – also diar-
  rhoea violent.
Cholera:   Cuprum – convulsive.
                Veratrum – cold sweat and vomiting.
                Camphor – extreme coldness – dry.
Where inflammation and discharges cease and convulsions come on.

**Mentals**
Delirium, confused. Always likes to be occupied. Bored if idle.

**Gastrointestinal**
Metallic taste (Cocculus, Mercurius, Natrum Carb, Rhus Tox.,
  Senega).
Eats *fast*. Desires cold food. Tendency to choke.

**Limbs**
Coldness of feet.
Cramps in the calves. Oil and copper rubbed on in multiple sclerosis;
  injections of Cuprum per Chamomilla for spasm of multiple sclerosis
  (special potency preparations).

Related to Proteus (bowel nosode).

## FERRUM METALLICUM

One of the four obesity remedies.
Palpitation, breathlessness, WEAKNESS EVEN AT REST.
Flushing of face on the least excitement, and yet cold.
CHILLY.
Pallid waxy. Anaemia.
PAINS are worse at rest, better from slow gentle motion (like Pulsatilla);
   better from heat, worse on rapid motion.
Muscles flabby and relaxed. Prolapse: rectum, vagina, bladder.
Distension of blood vessels, plethora, varicose veins, and haemorrhages
   – nose bleeds.
Effects of fluid loss like China.

**Mentals**
Sensitivity of nerves to pain. Restless, irritable, changeable in mood and
   impulsive.
Depression, anxiety, mental weariness. Upset by noise.

**Head**
Vertigo over water.
Congestive *headaches* better from pressure, worse on coughing.

**Respiratory**
Spasmodic cough, suffocative.

**Gastrointestinal**
Vomiting without much nausea – regurgitation of food.
Night vomiting. Diarrhoea on eating.
*Aversion* to meat, eggs, sour fruit.

**Rheumatic**
*Pains:* especially deltoid muscles, worse on motion, better slow moving,
better from heat. More often on the right side.

## GRAPHITES (Black Lead)

Chilly, pale, obese women, although a valuable remedy in skin eruptions
in men and women at all ages.

Sensitive also to a warm room, desire for open air.

Tendency to flush, and to nose bleeds.

SKIN ERUPTIONS often affect the bends of limbs, behind ears, scalp.
There is oozing thick honey-like exudate.

Itch may occur all over without eruption, skin hot in night.

Discharges are offensive. Psoriasis also with scaling.

Cicatrices and scars can be softened by this remedy.

### Mentals
Sad, despondent, lazy, .weeps easily especially at music, timid,
indecisive, apprehensive.

Extreme activity of mind in the evening and first part of the night,
keeping him awake.

### Eyes
The eyes are frequently affected with marked photophobia, pustular
inflammation, cysts and blepharitis with cracked, bleeding eyelids. (In
Sulphur the lids are always red.)

### Nose
Chronic nasal catarrh, with excoriation of nostrils, scabs and ulcers.

### Face
Cracks at corners of mouth, nails thick and distorted.

Cobweb sensation on the face.

Deafness – ear discharge. Hears better in a noise.

### Gastrointestinal
Duodenal ulcer pain relieved by food and drink, relieved by hot food
and warm milk, relieved by lying down.

Quite hungry, better from eating.

*Averse* to sweet, fish.

Constipation – knotty, lumpy stools with mucus or diarrhoea –
undigested, fetid.

## HEPAR SULPHURIS (Oyster Shell and Flowers of Sulphur)

HYPERSENSITIVENESS (to touch, pain, cold air), OFFENSIVENESS, IRRITABILITY.

### Generals

Aggravation from draught, putting his hand out of bed. (Silica is worse in wet cold weather, and better in warm, dry weather.)

Better in wet weather (warm wet).

Glands, swellings, *suppuration* but painful, sensitive even to breath of air or touch.

Sweats sour, offensive night and day – without relief.

Discharges offensive. Eruptions, moist, unhealthy, suppurating, sensitive.

Splinter-like pains. (Argentum Nit., Kali Carb., Nitric Acid, Silica.)

### Mentals

Hypersensitive and touchy, irritable, *impetuous*, anger out of proportion, discontented, grumbles, resents coming to the doctor, sudden murderous impulses.

### Eyes

Purulent eye discharge.

### Ears

Ear discharge, mastoid – offensive and *sensitive*.

### Respiratory

Suffocative cough, tightness (more than tickling) dry, deep cough – starts up wanting breath, worse on the *slightest-draught*. (Spongia – hoarse, difficult drawing breath – narrow larynx.)

Sweats with cough, weeps with or before cough, wheezing rattling and asthmatic. (Like Natrum Sulph. but it is worse in damp weather.)

### Stomach

Desires pickles and vinegar.

Mercurius, Hepar Sul. and Silica, if following one another, should be prescribed in this order.

IGNATIA (Seeds of St Ignatius Bean, containing strychnine)

The symptoms of Ignatia are PARADOXICAL, UNEXPECTED and PER-
VERSE. They are also changeable.
If the patient is in the chilly stage of a fever and is cold, he wants to be
uncovered.
When he is feverish and hot, he wants to be warm.
He is thirsty when cold and chilly, but not thirsty when feverish. The
more he coughs, the more the irritation makes him cough.
When a part is inflamed, it is relieved by hard pressure.
When the throat is inflamed he gets relief from swallowing solids.
In stomach complaints it is the simple unirritating foods which upset.
HYPERSENSITIVITY to pain.
Symptoms and pains are relieved by passing large quantities of urine.

## Generals
Chilliness – complaints worse in cold weather and out of doors, better
from sun, warmth, and clothing.
Rest relieves pains and movement worsens them; although hypersen-
sitive to pain, it is relieved by hard pressure.
Pains tend to occur in circumscribed spots (Kali Bich.).
There are cramps, spasms and twitching of muscles, especially on the
face.

## Mentals
Although both Nux Vomica and Ignatia have strychnine in them, the
Ignatia patient is seldom angry or violent. She is highly emotional,
capricious, moody and changeable. Sensitive, refined woman with
intuitive perception, quick to perceive, rapid in action.
   Rapid alternation of moods – gaiety alternates rapidly with melancholy and tearfulness, but not so self-pitying as Pulsatilla. Symptoms
often arise from sorrow at the loss of friends or from sympathy with the
troubles of others. The effects of GRIEF on sensitive natures often calls
for Ignatia – also mental anxiety and worry. These patients do not
resent attempts at consolation, which occurs in Natrum Mur. or Sepia.
Ignatia is a short-acting remedy in grief, and may need to be followed
by Natrum Mur. where there are long lasting effects and inability to
weep.

## Headaches
Appear suddenly and are severe – aggravated by noise and light, and
brought on by odours, especially tobacco. They are relieved by rest
and warmth, and lying on the painful side, and sometimes even by
stooping.

Pain like a nail being driven into the head (Thuja).
Headaches relieved by copious flow of urine (Gelsemium).

## Eyes
Photophobia and flashes and flickerings of light, but also conjunctivitis, lachrymation and blepharitis.

## Respiratory
Dry, hacking, spasmodic cough, paroxysmal – the more he coughs, the more the irritation makes him cough. Whooping cough.

## Gastrointestinal
Spasms in the throat, sensation of a lump better from swallowing solids.
Appetite capricious – either loss of appetite or craving for food. Cold food is preferred and there is dislike of alcohol, coffee, meat. Hiccough, vomiting and flatulence often emotional in origin.

## Genito-urinary
Copious urination which relieves headache.
*Dysmenorrhoea* – severe, cramping, labour-like pains with excessive flow and clotting, relieved by rest and by hard pressure. In the Ignatia type of woman.

## Extremities
Violent sudden neuralgias, with cramps and spasms.
Sciatica on any movement, better from rest, hard pressure, heat.

## Skin
Itching of the skin – often of value in the elderly with no evidence of skin eruption.

Natrum Mur. and Sepia follow well.

# IODUM

INTOLERANCE OF HEAT. Restlessness.
INORDINATE HUNGER with EMACIATION – only feels well when eating.
ENLARGEMENT OF GLANDS everywhere except mammary, which wither.
Dark haired, dark eyes, dark skin.

## Mentals
Anxious and restless, must be on the move (e.g. Arsenicum Alb., but this remedy is hot and Arsenicum Alb. is chilly.)
Impulses to violence, especially if still – hence he walks about, hurries, and gets exhausted with weakness.

## Respiratory
Excoriating catarrh, salivation.
Dry cough with stitches and burning, suffocative – all halogens (Bromine, Chlorine and Iodine) have irritation of mucous membranes, with rawness, inflammation or croup.
Cough worse in warm room.

## Gastrointestinal
Eructations, marked hunger better from eating.
Pains in the left hypochondrium and spleen.

## Other symptoms
Pains in joints at night in chronic arthritis.
Leucorrhoea yellow and corrosive.
Thyroid conditions, if other symptoms fit, with palpitation and feeling as if heart is squeezed (Lilium Tig.)

## KALI BICHROMICUM

This remedy has particular characteristics and local indications rather than a constitutional picture. It affects mucous membranes and skin and is characterised by ulceration, stringiness, yellowness and pain in spots. Complaints generally worse in hot weather. Rheumatic pains wander from joint to joint and alternate with other symptoms like catarrh.

THICK ROPY DISCHARGES, particularly from the nose, throat and bronchial tubes, but also in gastritis and leucorrhoea.

ULCERATION of the nasal septum (seen in chrome workers), crusts, dryness, obstruction of the nose and tendency to bleed. Pains at the root of the nose and in the sinuses – may relieve where there is sinus pain, and no discharge has come away.

ULCERATION of the throat and mouth – oedema of the uvula. Tongue is yellow and coated or glazed, red and cracked.

### Headaches
Blinding – sight returns as the headache intensifies, accompanied by dyspepsia. Violent headache aggravated by light, noise, better from warmth, pressure.

### Stomach
*Ulceration* of stomach, punched out, deep ulcers with emptiness, but easily filled (Lycopodium) wind and pain localised to a spot to the left of the xiphisternum. Vomiting sour and ropy mucus (sometimes in oesophageal diverticulum or hiatus hernia). Of use in the vomiting of drunkards.

### Other symptoms
*Ulceration* of the skin and legs; deep, punched out. Bone pain. Pains occur in distinct *spots* on the head or in the epigastrium. They tend to appear and disappear suddenly. There is *yellowness* of vision, yellow discharges, yellow watery vomitus.

Useful in measles where there are pustules on the cornea and pains extending from the throat to the ears, swollen salivary glands and catarrhal deafness.

## KALI CARBONICUM

Pale, soft, flabby-looking people, with sweat on the slightest exertion.
CHILLY, worse from cold, cold winds, cold applications (except piles).
Puffiness of upper eyelids.
General aggravation of symptoms between 2–4 a.m.
Symptoms often RIGHT SIDED.
STITCHING, CUTTING PAINS, WORSE at rest or on motion, from cold, pressure or lying on the affected side. (Bryonia better from rest, pressure.) These pains may affect the pleura, pericardium or joints, which are sensitive to pressure and touch. There is loss of elasticity and power in the ligaments and around the joints causing slackness and weakness. Pains are often present in the right outer thigh between the hip and knee. WEAKNESS of the BACK with pain, in old people or for years after a disc lesion or childbearing.

### Mentals
Drab, uninteresting people who tend to exaggerate symptoms, have a failure of will and inability to stand up to things, and hence keep returning frequently to the doctor. Irritable, hypersensitive, on edge, startled by noise and may cry out when startled or with pains. A sudden noise catches her 'in the stomach'. Never at peace, tries to do several jobs at once, and gets in a muddle. Fears to be alone, of the future, of dying or ghosts – imagination vivid.

### Headaches
Congestive over the right forehead and temple, severe and shooting, relieved by discharge of catarrh.

### Respiratory
A remedy with much catarrh, frothy or stringy. Frequently catching colds. Sensation of a splinter in the throat (Nitric Acid, Hepar Sulph.) or of a lump. Of value in whooping cough and in asthma, particularly when there is 3 a.m. aggravation and the patient must sit up and lean forward.

Right lower lobe pneumonia, with hard cough and then tough mucopurulent sputum, and the characteristic *stitching pains*.

### Heart
A potassium salt, and so we find a weak, irregular, intermittent pulse with low blood pressure.

### Gastrointestinal
Desire for *sweets* or sugar – takes too much starch.
Flabby tongue, thickly coated at the base.

Dyspepsia in the elderly – full bloated sensation, with wind in the bowels. In pyloric ulcer the pain comes on 2–3 hours after meals, with vomiting of stringy mucus.

Feels worse from eating, especially hot food – distension after eating.

Colic usually associated with gallbladder. (Colocynth has colic related to the bowel.) If colic keeps recurring in spite of Colocynth, try Kali Carb. Burning piles are relieved by cold application.

**Menses**
Profuse.

## LACHESIS (The Venom of the Surukuku or Bushmaster Snake)

This remedy is characterised by BLUENESS, the blue bloated face in cardiac failure, blueness of veins, or ulcers which bleed and heal poorly. Petechiae and ecchymoses. Valuable in severe sepsis or pneumonia and especially at the menopause. There are several characteristic symptoms.

There is an AGGRAVATION of all symptoms AFTER SLEEP, pains or asthma may wake her; afraid to go to sleep because she feels so ill on waking. Marked SENSITIVITY to TOUCH, CONSTRICTION of tight things especially round the neck, and to noise.

RELIEF from discharges, especially menstrual flow.

LEFT-SIDED symptoms – many of the Lachesis symptoms occur on the left side.

HEAT aggravates – faint in the heat, hot drinks aggravate, flushes marked.

Symptoms often OUT OF PROPORTION – sensations of choking, a lump or CONSTRICTION in the THROAT, are much more marked than the signs suggest. They are worse from touch, hot drinks, empty swallowing.

General aggravation of symptoms in the spring, and in mild, rainy, cloudy weather.

### Mentals

*Jealousy, suspicion* (thinks people are trying to poison her).

*Loquacity* – talks constantly, going off on to other lines of thought, but sometimes may be slow of speech and taciturn.

Religious insanity – feels wicked and full of sin.

Thinks she is under superhuman control and may be commanded to do things. Disturbance of time sense. Sensitive to noise.

### Headaches

Hammering or pulsating, often left-sided and worse from pressure and *after sleep.*

### Cardiac

Palpitation with fainting, cramp-like pains, dyspnoea, and quick, irregular pulse. Anginal pain.

### Gastrointestinal

Tongue trembles, is difficult to protrude, catches on the teeth. It is inflamed, swollen, painful – marked thirst.

Flatulence with intolerance of tight clothing, painful diarrhoea, spasms of the anus and large blue, bleeding piles.

**Genital**

A wonderful remedy in the menopause, where periods are suppressed or have stopped, or where there are flushes and palpitation and feelings of choking. Increased sexual desire at the menopause. Dysmenorrhoea with pains in the *left* ovary.

# LILIUM TIGRINUM

Usually fat and fair, poor colour.
HOT, HURRIED, WORRIED – rather like a hot Sepia, but Sepia has marked indifference.

## Mentals
Melancholy, silent, *depressed*, weepy.
Bad tempered, a bit aggressive, angry; exacting – things revolve round her. Feels she has something important to do, for which she alone is responsible, and no one else can do it, hence the hurry.
Full of fears – of going insane, of what happens after death, that she is suffering from a terrible disease.

## Headache
With ocular disturbance and muddled feeling, from mental strain, worse at the menses.

## Cardiac
Sensation as if the heart is '*grasped*' with palpitation – must bend double. (Opposite of Spigelia.)

## Gastrointestinal
Desire for heat (unlike Sepia). Hungry even after a good meal.
Sensitive in the epigastrium, cannot stand a belt round waist.
Pressure in the rectum and *constant desire* for stool.

## Genito-urinary
Pressure in the bladder with *constant desire* to urinate.
Sensation as if the whole *inside would fall out* through the vagina, not just the passive weight of Sepia but a forcible pressure.
Cannot stand, must sit down.
This *intense pressing down* in vagina, bladder and rectum is characteristic of Lilium Tigrinum. (The bearing down of Belladonna is better from standing. The bearing down of Pulsatilla is worse from lying, and better on moving.)
Uncontrollable sexual excitement with hurried feeling, worse before menses.
Menses heavy, clotting and irregular.

## LYCOPODIUM CLAVATUM (Club Moss)

This remedy comes from the spores of the club moss, which are inert until broken down by trituration, when an active ingredient is released. Lycopodium is indicated in patients who are pale, with a WORRIED FROWN, who look older than their years (prematurely grey). There is emaciation of the face and neck, with well-nourished body.

Often suited to intellectual people, with responsibilities – lawyers, accountants, doctors, ministers.

### Generals
Sensitive to *cold*, cold air, cold drinks, but headaches are worse from a
　　warm atmosphere.
Symptoms are often *right-sided* or go from right to left.
Aggravation 4–8 p.m.
*Worried frown* on forehead and *movements of the alae nasi*, especially
　　in pneumonia.

### Mentals
*Anticipatory* dread, fear of failure, aversion to undertaking new things, feeling of incompetence, and yet once he has started his speech or meeting he is capable and does well. Sensitive, emotional people, with anxious worried thoughts, weeps on meeting a friend or receiving a gift, sometimes despondent and gloomy.

Fears being alone, crowds, dark, death, ghosts and yet he does not want company, especially strangers. Wants someone in the house, but in the next room. Taciturnity because he does not wish to talk, forgetful, makes mistakes in words or writing.

### Headaches
Worse from heat, warmth of bed, lying down.
Better from cold, cold air, better from eating.

### Sore throats
Most marked on the right side, or going from right to left, better from
　　*warm* drinks.

### Respiratory
Catarrhal affections of eyes.
Nose blocked especially in infants, and then purulent discharge.
A remedy often indicated in pneumonia, especially on the right side,
　　with a dry teasing cough, anxious look, flapping nose, and
　　aggravation of symptoms or fever between 4–8 p.m.

**Gastrointestinal**

Frequently indicated in peptic ulcer, gastritis and liver and gallbladder complaints.

A very *flatulent* remedy (like China, Carbo Veg.) marked distension – must loosen her clothes, hungry and yet full up after a few mouthfuls. Wind in the bowel.

Desire for *sweet* food and *hot* drinks.

Aversion to meat, coffee. Upset by oysters.

Sour and acrid eructations.

Always worse from cold drinks and better from warm drinks.

Constipation without desire; also diarrhoea when other Lycopodium symptoms are present.

**Urinary**

Inactivity of the bladder with slow or feeble flow.

Deposits of red sand in the urine. Enuresis, and polyuria in the night.

**Genital**

A remedy often indicated in impotency, especially if this follows overindulgence in sexual activities for some years previously.

Neuralgic pains in the right ovary, dryness of the vagina, delayed or suppressed menses.

**Limbs**

Restlessness and rheumatic pains relieved by motion, and by the warmth of the bed.

One foot hot, the other cold, numbness of the limbs.

Burning sensation between the scapulae.

**MEDORRHINUM** (Nosode made from urethral discharge containing gonococci – being potentised it is safe, and does not actually contain these organisms)

A remedy of value in catarrhal conditions, ASTHMA, leucorrhoea and ARTHRITIS. It helps the general health and development of mongols. The person requiring this remedy tends to be plump, with wide nose, full lips and much hair, coarse and with bushy eyebrows. There is a tendency to have dandruff and tumours, sebaceous cysts, moles and warts. (The Sycotic type.) Several other characteristics are present. Symptoms often BETTER at the SEA. (Asthma, rheumatism.)

Generally WORSE during the DAY or 3–5 a.m. (Syphilinum worse at night.) DAMP weather relieves but cold weather aggravates. BURNING FEET.

## Mentals
Hypersensitive, dislikes being touched or people around him.
Easily fatigued; aware of this and *hurries* in order to complete something before weariness and depression overtake him.
Physical *restlessness*, cannot keep still, fidgets.
Anxiety over the future, worries, depressed even suicidal, selfish, fear of dying, one of the *anticipatory* remedies.
Difficulty expressing himself, loss of words, muddled, tendency to exaggerate.
Clairvoyance, sensation of *unreality* (as if outside of himself), time seems to pass slowly, and therefore he is disinclined to work or make any exertion.

## Headache
Right frontal. Vertigo better from lying down. (Conium worse on lying.)

## Respiratory
Catarrh, sinusitis, bronchitis.
*Asthma* relieved by lying in the *knee-elbow position*, with the face on the pillow (a strange symptom of great value in selecting this remedy). Remember also amelioration *at the sea.*

## Gastrointestinal
Desires *salt*, sweet, sour, pickles, iced things.
Abdominal pains better from lying on the abdomen.
Green, irritating stools in babies.
Must *lean back* to pass a stool. Oozing from anus.

**Menses**
Profuse, leucorrhoea which stains the clothing, sterility.

**Urinary**
Often of value in *enuresis*.

**Rheumatic**
*Arthritis* better at the sea, worse during the day, with sensitive vertebrae and lumbar stiffness. Pains in the heels. Damp weather relieves but cold aggravates.

## MERCURIUS SOLUBILIS (Black Oxide of Mercury)

Mercury is well known for its former use in the treatment of syphilis, and yet in fact there are many resemblances between the features of syphilis and the toxic effects of mercury. Possibly some of the action of the drug was homoeopathic in this disease.

The characteristic symptoms indicating Mercurius are: Sensitivity to CHANGES of temperature – aggravation from all forms of HEAT, especially the heat of the bed, but also from cold, open air or wet and damp.

Aggravation of symptoms at NIGHT.
Profuse SWEATING without relief.
Creeping chilliness in the early stages of a cold or fever.
Foulness of the mouth, with offensive breath. SALIVATION.

### Respiratory
Throat raw and smarting, with exudate or ulceration. The *tongue* is flabby, coated yellow or white, moist and shows the imprint of the teeth round its edge.
*Salivation* with thirst and moist tongue, offensive breath.
The teeth are decayed or black, the gums spongy and bleeding, and toothache is frequent. Metallic taste.
Thick green or yellow discharge from the nose with raw nostrils.
Otitis media in measles may be helped by Mercurius.
The *right* lower lobe of the lung is usually involved in pneumonia, and the patient feels *worse lying on the right side.*

### Gastrointestinal
Desire for stimulants, preference for liquid rather than solid, and as mentioned thirst and *salivation*.
There is sensitivity in the liver region, worse from lying on the right side.
Acute colitis, and frequently indicated in dysentery or ulcerative colitis with slimy, bloody stools with colic and fainting and *marked tenesmus*, continuing after stool (can hardly leave the toilet the urge is so marked – here Mercurius Corrosivus is usually better).
Also may be constipated with hard, knotty stools and mucus.

### Genito-urinary
Nephritis, irritation at the end of the penis, nocturnal erections and increased desire, but great debility. Ulcers of the penis (Syphilis).
Sweat of external genitalia.
Excessive periods, leucorrhoea profuse, excoriating and worse at night.

**Skin**
Eruptions of all kinds, papular, pustular, urticarial and chronic ulcers.

**Other symptoms**
Inflammatory *rheumatism* with swelling of joints worse from heat of
  the bed but also on uncovering. Bone pains worse at night.
Always the sweating and chilliness of Mercurius.
*Tremor* of the hands and tongue.
Great debility of body and mind.

There are few mental symptoms associated with Mercurius, but they
may have marked restlessness, and a feeling of hurry and anxiety. In
severe illness they may develop slowness in answering, poor memory
and even paralysis, spasms and cramps.
   In diphtheria Mercurius Cyanatus is almost specific.

## NATRUM MURIATICUM

Pale, greasy skin, tendency to acne, emaciation in spite of eating, flushed on excitement.

These patients are reticent and nervous, and need to summon up courage to come to the doctor. Once there, they are deliberate, covering their nervousness with a self-assured appearance, but showing tremor in their movements.

### Generals

Worse from heat, better in the open air, but can be chilly. Worse at the *seaside*, but sometimes better with the sea air; aggravation from thunder.

Intermittent fevers with chill but worse from heat. Thirst for cold during chill. Periodicity.

*Desires: salt*, fish.

*Aversion:* fat, bread, rich food, meat, coffee.

### Mentals

Effects of grief or love affair; weepy feeling but cannot cry, yet weeps if consoled. Reticent, broods, harbours resentment, hates sympathy, but likes attention due to him. Not good at mixing. Sensitive to noise, music; startled easily.

Claustrophobia. Impatient. Poor sense of humour – tends to laugh when he should be solemn.

Instability (moods up and down), takes up with people and drops them. Nice to know, but difficult to live with.

Sleep disturbed by unpleasant thoughts.

### Head

Headaches are hammering with zig-zags in vision; may wake with headache. Sensitive to noise. Headaches midday to evening, especially in sun. Vision tends to give out on reading, eyes sore and tired, watery eyes in wind.

### Respiratory

Coryza – thick white, but with dryness of mucous membranes, frequent colds, inflamed nose.

### Gastrointestinal

Empty about 11 a.m. May eat much but remains thin.

Mapped tongue.

Constipation – dry, crumbling stool.

**Genito-urinary**
Menses delayed – feels worse at menses, not before it – backache.
Slow urination – cannot pass urine in presence of others.

**Skin**
Gluey, moist eruptions, itchy, exfoliating.
Herpes, crack centre of lower lip, painful spots on nose or chin, acne along hair margin.

**Back**
Vertebrae sensitive, yet relieved by lying on something hard.

A remedy often useful in nervous and emotional states, thyrotoxicosis, palpitation. Long acting. Bryonia is the acute of Natrum Mur. – use Bryonia in the acute phase of headache and follow up with Natrum Mur. Apis and Ignatia are also related remedies.

## NATRUM SULPHURICUM (Sodium Sulphate, Glauber's Salts)

This remedy is most valuable in cases of asthma, rheumatism and diarrhoea, and after head injury.

It is a Sycotic remedy with warts, condylomata, catarrhal conditions and marked aggravation in damp and cold, or near the sea. Symptoms are also worse in warm, wet weather. (Lachesis, Carbo Veg., Silica.) Sensitive to warm atmosphere, better in the open air.

### Periodicity
Worse in the Spring. (Lachesis, Rhus Tox.)
Worse 4–5 a.m. – especially cough and asthma.
2–3 a.m. colic.
Diarrhoea *after* rising in the morning.

### Mentals
Depressed, tearful, irritable in the morning, full of anxiety, sensitive to *small* noises; music makes her sad or annoys her.
Fear of the future, tired of life but does not really want to kill herself. (Aurum may commit suicide.)
Dislikes to speak or be spoken to. Mental exertion causes headache.

### Headaches
Occipital, especially after *head injury*. May also have loss of memory, twitchings and even epilepsy after head injury.
Salivation with headache.

### Respiratory
Catarrhal – *greenish discharges* everywhere, nose, sputum, leucorrhoea.
Loose cough with pains and soreness of the chest – must hold his sides with his hands. Sputum green and salty. (Bryonia – dry cough.)
Feeling of oppression of the chest aggravated by damp.
Asthma worse from damp, at 4–5 a.m., and from sea air.
Left basal pneumonia with pains as above.

### Gastrointestinal
Dragging and pains in the liver, bilious vomiting, nausea, eructations, flatulence and rumbling in the bowels. Colic 2–3 a.m.
Cannot digest starch, milk, potatoes.
Diarrhoea in the morning *after rising*. (Sulphur. Diarrhoea forces him out of bed.)

**Rheumatic**

Rheumatic pains and rheumatoid arthritis, especially worse in damp and cold. There is restlessness like Rhus but also aggravation from motion as in Bryonia.

Complementary to Arsenicum, Thuja.

## NITRIC ACID

Tend to be dark-haired with brown eyes.
Great debility and lack of stamina of all the acids.
A CHILLY patient with profuse sweat of hands and feet.
Tendency to WARTS, ulceration, fissures, bleeding, offensiveness.
SPLINTER-like pains – in bone, throat, nose, anus.
General aggravation from WIND, thunder, WET.

### Mentals
These patients are depressed and despairing, anxious and yet
   *indifferent*. Irritable, intolerant of sympathy.
Suspicious, obstinate and restless. The irritability, especially in
   children, is improved by travelling.
Sensitive to noise, pain, touch and jar.
Fear of death. (In some respects like Sepia, but Sepia loathes fat and
   does not like salt.)

### Headache
Fullness in the head, and a sensation of a tight bandage around the head
– sensitive to touch.

### Respiratory
Nasal catarrh, acrid and excoriating the upper lip; nostrils ulcerated.
   *Cracks* at the corners of the mouth.
There is splinter-like pain in the throat on swallowing.
Offensive salivation like Mercurius.
Inflammation of the lungs.

### Gastrointestinal
Dirty mouth as described.
Desire for *fat* and *salt*, (like Sulphur), even although fat may disagree.
Orifices tend to be affected, mouth, nose, anus, vulva. Anal *fissures* and
   piles – very painful, sharp and splinter-like pain lasting for hours
   after stool, even a soft stool. (Nux Vomica pain is better after stool
   and the pain in Mercurius lasts all the time.)

### Genito-urinary
Inflammation and ulceration of the vulva and warty growths.
Urine with strong offensive smell like a horse's. The urine feels cold as it
   is passed.

## NUX VOMICA

Persons of anxious, zealous, fiery temperament, offended at the harmless word or malicious and IRRITABLE, with anger and violence or desire to kill. They hate contradiction, are troubled by little things, must attend to details, fastidious. Cannot sleep as business affairs crowd upon them. May fall asleep after 3 a.m., and wake with bad taste and headache. They worry over others, and may be sullen and quiet and averse to doing things. It is a remedy for indiscretion of eating or drinking or overdoing things, work, stress.

### Generals
*Chilly* persons, worse in *dry* or windy weather, from draughts and yet dislikes stuffy atmosphere.

Burning heat with red face in fever but cannot move or uncover without feeling chilly.

*Sensitive* to smells, noise, pain.

Spasms and convulsions made worse by the slightest touch on the head.

### Headache
Dull headache in the morning after overeating or overdrinking, or when under stress.

Occipital headache in morning.

Headache associated with indigestion or liver upset.

### Respiratory
Profuse coryza from one nostril, with obstruction.

Raw throat and larynx.

Early morning cough, violent and causing headache.

### Gastrointestinal
*Desire* for tasty food, fat, rich food which upsets.

Flush and fainting while eating, aggravation from meat.

Nausea with *much retching*, difficult to empty stomach.

Pregnancy sickness with sleeplessness. Liver congestion.

Dirty brown posterior half of tongue.

Distension and indigestion 2–3 hours after food.

Spasmodic constipation – with *ineffectual urging*, and sensation of incomplete stool with much straining and piles.

Colicky diarrhoea with nausea, hard lumps with watery stool, mucus and urging.

Also ineffectual urging to urinate.

Antidote to Sulphur.

## OPIUM

Remember the opposite effects of overdose – first sensations of physical and mental happiness, stimulation and overexcitability and then gradually stuporose. Opium is one of the few drugs which does NOT cause pain in its provings.

LOSS OF MORAL SENSE, lying and thieving – or, in children, lack of development of moral sense.

PAINLESSNESS – ulcers that are painless.

INACTIVITY and torpor – PARALYSIS – leading to the typical picture of the stroke patient.

Unconscious, stertorous respiration, jaw dropped, pupils contracted, face mottled, purple, hot with sweat, cheeks blowing out, and paralysis – no response.

INACTIVITY of bowel, symptomless constipation.

Inactivity of bladder – retention with full bladder.

AILMENTS from FRIGHT – where fear remains long after.

OPPOSITES: We can also see sleeplessness, anxiety, increased sensitivity to noise – can hear 'flies walking on the wall'. Delirium, eyes wide open, face red, puffed up. Vivid imagination, irritable, easily frightened.

Twitchings, jerkings, convulsions – in this situation he needs to be uncovered – wants cool air.

Bed feels too hot – wants to move to a cool place or be uncovered.

Failure of the patient to react to the indicated remedy would suggest the need for Opium.

## PHOSPHORUS

The Phosphorus patient is usually tall and slim, either with dark hair, brown eyes and long eyelashes, and the pallor or pink and white complexion of those with a tendency to tuberculosis, or red-haired with freckles and a lively sensitive disposition. Constitution feeble with liability to catch colds and coughs, suffer from bowel or liver complaints and to bleed easily. Profuse sweats on exertion or in bed in the morning – sweat on the upper lip on exertion or mental effort. Bruises and bleeds easily, menses profuse, bright red.

### Generals
*Chilly* patients.
Symptoms of the head and stomach are better from cold.
Symptoms of the chest and limbs are better from heat.
So we find the headaches are worse in heat and a warm room, and
    better from cold applications and from sleep.

### Mentals
Indifference to loved ones, apathy, answers slowly, great sense of fatigue, disinclination to work. Unlike Sepia, Phosphorus patients crave sympathy, company, touch, stroking; need reassurance.

Anxious, restless, full of fears – of thunderstorm, dark, death, that something will happen; full of strange imaginings – vivid imagination in children. Artistic, extrovert, musical and often untidy. Attractive, sensitive people. Sleep helps – always better from even a short sleep.

### Respiratory
Frequently indicated in chest infections. Hard, dry, tight cough, which
    racks the patient, husky rough voice worse in the evening (Causticum
    in morning).
Cough worse lying on the left side, worse going from warm to cold air,
    from talking or laughing.
Sputum salty, bloody. Right lower lung often affected in pneumonia.
    Thirst for cold drinks.

### Gastrointestinal
Stomach symptoms of vomiting, burning or bleeding are relieved by cold drinks, which are vomited after being warmed up in the stomach. Weak, empty sensation with desire to eat, and burning in the back between the scapulae. *Desire* for *salt,* tasty food, sour and spicy, and craving for *ice cold drinks* and icecream. Chronic loose stools with profuse diarrhoea and loss of anal control. Sometimes bloody mucus and tenesmus, or long slim, hard, dry stools difficult to pass. (Of value in colitis.)

## PHYTOLACCA DECANDRA (Poke Weed)

This remedy is like Mercurius in many respects, especially in its throat and mouth symptoms.

It affects skin, throat, fibrous and osseous tissues, breasts. Symptoms worse at NIGHT, on COLD days, in cold damp weather, in a cold room, but also worse from the HEAT OF THE BED. Pains are SHOOTING – electric shocks worse on motion and at night, desire to move but aggravation from motion.

### Throat

Dry, rough fauces and pharynx, congested, *dark red* (Belladonna: bright red). Hot feeling like a ball of red hot iron. Swallowing difficult and painful – pain shoots to ears. Regurgitation from nostrils, inability to swallow even water. Ulceration of mouth and throat. Irresistible inclination to bite teeth together. Worse from cold in all things *except* the throat, which is *worse from hot.*

### Mammary Gland

Mastitis – painful, inflamed, hot, unbearable, sore nipples with fissures.
Also indurated sore lumps, worse in cold damp. In nursing mothers, and
    also chronic mastitis, often troublesome during menses.
Of value also in cows with this condition.

### Rheumatic

*Rheumatic* pains, burning, shooting worse at night and in damp
    weather.
Inflammation of fibrous sheaths.
Pains fly like electric shocks, especially in deltoid attachment.
Shooting pain in right shoulder joint with stiffness and aching along the
    trapezius.
Tension and pressure in the parotid region – periarticular rheumatism.
Stiff neck: pain on the slightest movement (where Bryonia and Rhus
    Tox. fail).

# PLATINA

## Mentals
The characteristic symptoms which make us think of Platina in a patient are *arrogance*, an overwhelming pride in self and contempt for others. They feel superior and look down on others – this loss of sense of proportion is also present in a physical sense too – things around them appear small.

Often the patient *desires to injure*, physically or mentally, those they love most. This may result in hysterical women from fright, shock or prolonged excitement. The patient may feel deeply wounded and almost paranoid.

There are *alternating* extremes, hilarity and anger, wretchedness and excitement following one another quite quickly.

Fear of death or that something will happen.

## Headaches
Of gradual onset accompanied by numbness of the scalp and resulting from emotional causes, particularly sexual excitement or at the menstrual period.

## Gastrointestinal
Flatulence, colic and constipation. The stool is clay-like and adherent with much straining. There is a sensation of retraction of the abdomen at the navel, like that occurring in Plumbum.

## Genital
Symptoms in this region are often marked in this remedy. There is extreme sensitivity and hyperaesthesia of the genitalia. Increased sexual desire with sometimes masturbation and nymphomania.

Pain over the left ovary, and heavy periods.

## Other symptoms
Pains generally come and go gradually. There is a feeling of numbness accompanying pain.

Sensation of constriction like a band round a limb.

Predominantly a female remedy, but not entirely so.

## PLUMBUM (Lead)

This remedy has certain characteristic indications.

HYPERAESTHESIA, with extreme sensitivity to touch with LOSS OF POWER. This occurs in acute conditions. Where there is more chronic paralysis and weakness, sensation is also lost.

EMACIATION and MUSCLE WASTING.

PARALYSIS chiefly of the extensors, upper limb from the centre to the periphery (wrist drop). The paralysis is first local and then general with difficulty in articulation or in passing urine, and coldness.

A remedy of value in progressive muscular atrophy (Hughes).

RETRACTION of parts. Violent abdominal pain with retraction of the abdomen and pain as if the umbilicus is pulled back to the spine. (Platina.)

### Mentals

Indifference, depression, drowsiness and melancholy.

Although intelligent, the intellect is slowed – *slow* to remember, *slow* to answer, *slow* to react to pain (in chronic cases).

Hysterical, changeable, inclination to *deceive* – the patient may give a completely false impression of his home circumstances. Anxious sighing.

Encephalopathy with headache, visual disturbances and fits.

### Gastrointestinal

Abdominal pain as described above with retraction of the abdomen.

Obstructive symptoms with faintness and cold sweat. *Constipation with colic.* The colic is relieved by firm pressure.

Excessive thirst.

Blue line on the gums (poisoning).

### Urinary

Chronic infections, with mucus and albuminuria.

### Spasms

Neuralgic cramps, rectal spasm.

Feeling of a tight band round the leg. (Platina.)

### PSORINUM (Seropurulent Matter from Scabies Vesicle)

This remedy has similarities to Sulphur, but is characterised by marked chilliness and dislike of open air.

LACK OF VITAL REACTION – slowness of digestion, in passing stool or urine.

FOULNESS OF DISCHARGES, offensive breath, stools, leucorrhoea, eruptions.

### Generals
*Chilly.* Generally worse in the open air or from draughts.

Skin symptoms often predominate. The skin is rough and dry, ichthyotic, with fissures, cracks and bleeding. Many types of eruption but usually *offensive*, oozing – pimples, boils, crusts, vesicles.

*Eczema* – very itchy and worse from warmth.

Scratches until raw. Worse at night. Better from cool air. This contrasts with the general aggravation from cold and open air.

### Mentals
Depressed, hopeless, despair of recovery, thinks his business will fail. Irritable, wants to be alone. Hates to be *washed*. Feelings of guilt, as if he has committed a great sin.

### Headaches
Violent, throbbing, periodic, frontal – must cover the head (Silica). Better after breakfast or eating. Must get up in the night to eat.

### Eyes
Eyelids thickened and red.

### Ears
Ears – eczema, scabs – also brownish, offensive pus.

### Respiratory
Frequent colds with constantly running nose – very useful in hayfever, but also thick yellow discharge.

Dirty throat with mucus.

Asthma – cannot breathe in the open air, wants to go home and lie down. *Lies flat on the back,* with arms outspread. This is an unusual and valuable symptom.

### Gastrointestinal
Hunger but nausea. Eructations like rotten eggs.

Stools watery, brown, *offensive*. Hastiness, urging (like Sulphur), flatulence (like Aloes), and difficulty in expelling soft stool (Alumina, China, Nux Moschata).

## Other peculiar symptoms
Sick babies fret and worry and scream at night.

Patient often feels *unusually well,* the day before or shortly prior to an attack (of asthma, diarrhoea or skin eruption).

During fever, patient is very hot and *sweating* profusely.

He also sweats with some relief after an acute illness, but is slow to recover.

Cannot bear limbs to touch one another (even fingers).

## PULSATILLA (The Pasque Flower)

This remedy is often thought of as a remedy for women and girls, and so it is, but some men also fit the symptom picture. Frequently fair with blue eyes, tendency to be plump.

### Generals
Pulsatilla is always *worse in a warm atmosphere,* and yet can be chilly in a warm room.

Better in *open air,* cold dry air (worse wet), better for *slow movement;* worse in the *evening.*

*Changeable* – in temperament, stools, rheumatic pains.

One-sided sweat of the face.

### Mentals
Slow and phlegmatic, of a mild, yielding, tearful disposition. They laugh and cry easily. Like sympathy, but do not give it as easily as Phosphorus; they are also suspicious, jealous and irritable and peevish (not violent), touchy, feel slighted. Imagines certain foods are not good for her. Dwells on religious notions and thinks she has sinned.

Fear of dark, alone, ghosts – of opposite sex; aversion to marriage.

A baby has a pitiful cry – wants caress (Chamomilla – a snarling cry; wants spanking).

### Vertigo
With nausea, worse in warm room, using eyes, lying down.

### Headaches
Worse in a hot room, using eyes; better in cool air, during motion.

Worse at menstrual period.

### Ears
Otitis media or bland discharge.

### Face
Eyes sore, red, itchy, styes. Crack in middle of lower lip.

### Respiratory
*Catarrh* of all kinds, yellow or green, *bland,* better in open air, sinusitis, bad smell in the nose, with discharge, crusts, bleeding. Loss of taste and smell. Hayfever in a Pulsatilla patient. Cough dry in evening, loose in morning.

### Gastrointestinal

Desires sweet, may like tasty foods which upset; fat and rich pastries disagree.

Sour vomiting and eructations – mouth foul in morning.

*Absence of thirst* even with a dry mouth or during a fever. Likes ice-cream but it upsets if taken when patient is warm. Better from cold food and drink.

Bloated and distended – slow to digest.

Stools changeable, green, constipation with urging without stool.

Haemorrhoids worse lying still, better on gentle motion.

### Genito-urinary

Frequent, scanty urine with urging. Lying on back causes desire to urinate. Involuntary urination from coughing, laughing, enuresis. Menses late or absent, scanty, intermittent and changeable, with colicky pain – suppressed after getting wet. Dragging down sensations (like Sepia). Leucorrhoea may be bland like other Pulsatilla discharges but can be excoriating. Puffiness and swelling relieved by flow.

Strong sexual desire in male and female (in spite of mental fear of opposite sex).

### Sleep

Cannot sleep till late on in night; dreams of cats; sleeps with hands over head.

### Skin

Skin is hot, dislikes many clothes. Small brown patches of psoriasis or measles-like rash; also purplish spots (like Lachesis).

### Limbs

Congestion of limbs, varicose veins, chilblains, hot feet in bed.

### Rheumatic

Rheumatism moves about from joint to joint, always changeable but better cool.

Pains in limbs worse from hanging down. (Vipera.)

Often indicated in measles with the typical rash, sore eyes, photophobia, cough and catarrh and tendency to ear and chest complications.

Frequently useful in asthma or the recurring coughs of children.

Mumps, especially when male develops orchitis.

## RHUS TOXICODENDRON (The great rheumatic remedy, also of value in skin eruptions)

Rheumatic HEADACHE, feels sore in muscles, caused by draught or DAMP, especially occiput, worse bending head backwards.

Rheumatic IRITIS from exposure to WET – pains shoot through the eyes to the back of the head, worse at night. Orbital cellulitis.

Paralysis of eye muscles from exposure to cold and WET. Pain in maxillary joints, cracking.

Stiffness and pain in neck and back, aching in SMALL of back. Strain of left shoulder joint – pains in joint and arm, aching and numbness. Articular inflammation.

Pains in wrists and hands.

Dull aching right sciatic nerve. Stiffness in knees and feet. Aching in legs, unable to rest for a moment.

Paroxysmal pains from getting wet.

The pains of Rhus Tox. are worse on first moving but relieved by continued movement. (Rhododendron pain is relieved immediately on moving.)

Stiffness of part on FIRST MOVING.

Aggravation from draught, first movement, cold, wet, at rest.

Amelioration heat and when warmed by exercise.

RESTLESSNESS. Must move the part. Pains worse AT NIGHT.

Numbness and twitching of extremities; traumatic paralysis.

Alternation with Bryonia, as symptoms change.

FEVERS: with restlessness, delirium, suspicion of being poisoned. (Influenza, paratyphoid.)

Dryness of the mouth with great thirst; red triangular tip of the tongue.

Effects of OVEREXERTION of a group of muscles, or over-use of the voice, which is initially hoarse and then improves with movement.

### Skin

Eruptions which are *vesicular* or pustular or even erysipelatous.

Eczema of palms and fingers, blistering eruptions of the vulva and *shingles*. Herpes of the lips.

# SEPIA

Sepia tends largely to be a female remedy, although occasionally we come across a male Sepia. She is thin, sallow with freckles or pigmentation and often a butterfly eruption across the nose and cheeks (like Rosacea). She has a dull, slow, stupid appearance, and yet can become vivacious, gay and sensitive, especially after exercise or dancing, which she loves. She complains of tiredness, weakness and dragging down sensations as if a prolapse may occur – she must sit down and cross her legs. She has low backache which is better from pressure and from active exercise.

## Generals
*Chilly* with cold feet, but flushes easily and sweats in axillae, back and genital region.
Faint on standing or kneeling and in a hot atmosphere.
Usually better from sleep. (Phosphorus)

## Mentals
The characteristic of Sepia is a loss of interest and indifference, particularly to loved ones. She is irritable, weepy and cannot cope – wants to get away from things. She is averse to sympathy and yet dreads solitude, weeps on telling symptoms or at music, and is helped by a good cry. She is usually tidy, but cannot be bothered; resents neighbours who try to help. Sensitive to noise; fear of incurable disease, insanity or poverty. Always better from active exertion or dancing, when she becomes alive.

## Gastrointestinal
*Desires:* Tasty, spicy food, vinegar.
*Aversion:* Fat, meat, milk.
Empty feeling relieved by eating, but nausea at the smell of food or tobacco (pregnancy sickness).
Constipation with fullness or ball in rectum – cannot expel stool and may have prolapse of rectum.

## Head
Headache often associated with nausea and relieved by sleep.

## Genital
Irregularity of menses, too early or too late. Premenstrual tension, heavy period with only slight relief from the flow. Burning leucorrhoea. May be of value in sterility.

## Skin
Vesicular eruptions, herpes, warty lesions on the neck, and of course, the sallow appearance and tendency to butterfly eruption.

## SILICA
A remedy often of value where there is sepsis, lack of reaction, failure to heal; for expulsion of splinters and pus in chronic lesions; induration of glands, especially parotids, fistulae. Tuberculosis.

Small neat people, with dull, lifeless hair; children have a big head and small body.

### Generals
*Chilly:* pale – 'dead hands' relieved by hot bathing.

Rough, cracked lips, fissures at the corners of the mouth, nails rough and yellow and poor quality.

Cold clammy feet and hands, profuse *sweats* of head and *feet* which are offensive.

Symptoms occur in cold damp weather.

### Mentals
Lack of strength (not necessarily of 'guts'), exhausted by talking, and therefore, shy and dislikes talking to people.

*Resentful,* overconscientious, but witty and good fun if brought out. Lack of confidence. *Dread of failure.*

Irritable, especially in the morning; child is cross and cries if spoken to. Anticipation upsets.

### Headache
Better from heat, wrapping up. Pain from occiput extending to right eye.

Worse from cold, exertion, physical and mental.

### Eyes
Inflammation of eyes, lashes fall out, crusting lids, blocked lachrymal duct.

### Respiratory
Catarrh of ears, discharge offensive, yellow. Chronic recurring sore throats. Suffocative rattling cough worse from cold or draught. Colds tend to settle in the chest.

### Gastrointestinal
Likes cold food and drink; aversion to and upset by hot drinks or food, which makes him sweat.

*Milk* upsets (Natrum Carb.). Recurring bilious vomit. Failure to assimilate (like Gaertner).

Constipation – lack of push – the stool slips back; offensive stools.

### Sleep
Sleepless – wakes, thinks and worries and finally drops off, but feels better with even a short sleep.

Silica is the chronic of Pulsatilla.

## STANNUM METALLICUM

Persons growing feeble over a long period; increasing weakness, cachexia, catarrhal conditions and neuralgia.

Sensitive to pain, increasing aversion to work, in business or at home; always tired.

Sallow complexion.

Great weariness, exhaustion on talking, weakness of the larynx and chest.

### Neuralgia
Gradual onset, increasing, gradually diminishing. (Pulsatilla: gradual onset and sudden let up. Belladonna: sudden onset with intensity at once, ceases suddenly.) Usually in the morning.

### Sensitive
To cold, and every change of weather.

### Headache
Every morning over one eye, especially left, spreading over forehead increasing gradually and decreasing gradually, and often with vomiting.

### Respiratory
Colds go to the chest – prone to tuberculosis.

Racking cough with retching; copious thick green, *sweetish* sputum. Coughs this up easily but more remains.

Weakness of the voice; hoarseness; talking makes him feel weak. Empty feeling in the chest, dyspnoea.

Rawness in the trachea. Paroxysms of cough, worse on talking, singing, laughing, lying on the side and from warm drink.

### Gastrointestinal
Constipation; hard, dry stools, urging but cannot pass stool, which may be soft. Colic better doubling up.

### Genital
In women a history of violent abdominal neuralgia, but once it goes she has a thick yellow-green leucorrhoea.

Menses early and profuse; feelings of prolapse.

## STAPHISAGRIA

This plant remedy has as its chief characteristic the mental picture. Almost all its complaints are a result of SUPPRESSED INDIGNATION, PENT UP WRATH, and RESENTMENT. The patient becomes very angry but keeps it in and then occasionally will let go and throw objects about. This anger can lead to headache, colic, rheumatic and joint pains. Takes offence easily. In adolescents with an unhappy love affair (like Natrum Mur.). As a result of this anger the patient trembles, loses his voice and cannot work or concentrate, becomes sleepless and develops headache. There is great indifference and weakness of memory. Symptoms also develop as a result of sexual excesses, or dwelling too much on sexual subjects. It is also of value in intense, energetic people with pride and envy (like Platina).

The other characteristic is SENSITIVITY, particularly to pain, with marked AGGRAVATION FROM TOUCH. Inflamed parts are very sensitive (like Hepar Sulph.), but there is also sensitivity to noise, tastes, odours. Decaying teeth in children are exquisitely tender.

It is indicated in the pain of INCISED WOUNDS or stretching operations (rectal or gynaecological).

### Headache
Numb, dull pain in the occiput or forehead with pains pressing inwards and outwards, especially resulting from indignation, and aggravated by *touch*.

### Eyes
A remedy for blepharitis, styes and nodosities or cysts of the eyelids. The eyes often appear sunken.

### Gastrointestinal
Colic resulting from anger (like Colocynth and Chamomilla).
Diarrhoea and colic from eating or drinking.
Haemorrhoids very sensitive.

### Genito-urinary
Irritable bladder with urging for days after pent up anger. A curious symptom of burning when *not* urinating and less when actually passing urine. Cystitis after first intercourse (honeymoon cystitis due to stretching). Increased sexual desire in both sexes with impotence in the male, and shooting pain in the ovary and irregular menses in the female.

Condylomata and warts especially round the anus or genitals.

**Skin**

Crusting, oozing, itching eruptions of the scalp, again very sensitive to touch.

Chronic induration of glands.

**Rheumatic**

Pains, arthritis and nodosities (arthritic or gouty), with stiffness and sense of fatigue in all the joints all worse from *touch*. Nightly bone pains. Pains particularly occurring as a result of anger, indignation or resentment, or accompanied by these, as often in cases of rheumatoid arthritis.

## SULPHUR

This remedy is often thought of as a skin remedy, but it also covers many conditions in patients with characteristic sulphur general symptoms. It is Hahnemann's great antipsoric remedy.

BURNING, REDNESS, OFFENSIVENESS, DIRTINESS.

These patients often have a rough, dry, scaly skin, which breaks and suppurates. Skin lesions of all kinds, itchy, burning, worse from heat or bathing.

Boils, abscesses, severe acne, eczema, dermatitis, psoriasis.

BURNINGS in all organs, hands and feet worse from heat. PERIODICITY – every 7 days.

REDNESS of orifices – lips, nose, anus, vulva. Eyelids red, crusty, itchy.

OFFENSIVE discharges which excoriate and burn. Congestion, varicose veins and ulcers.

Sulphur patients are HOT and aggravated by heat, but can feel cold and dislike wet and cold wet weather. Hot feet which they put out of bed. Generally worse from STANDING, after SLEEP, after eating.

The typical Sulphur patient is lean, lank, stoop-shouldered, dirty and untidy (this latter may only be of one article of clothing, e.g. tie or jersey inside out), but some are stout, plethoric and cheerful. Children often look dirty and have coarse reddish hair – dislike bathing.

### Mentals
They are often introspective, selfish (thinking of themselves), argumentative. They have an aversion to work, cannot concentrate and tend to theorise or have a philosophical outlook. (This may occur during illness in an otherwise hard-working person.) In spite of their mess, and offensive discharges and odour, they are very sensitive to bad odours – smell of their own stools. They see beauty in ordinary things.

### Headaches
Congestive like a band round the head, or pressure and heat on the vertex. Worse on stooping but better from warmth (unusual in Sulphur – opposite of Arsenicum).

Dizziness, especially on standing, or rising in the morning.

### Respiratory
Chronic *catarrh* with dirty nose and irritating discharge from nostrils with redness. Ears may discharge or are itchy and deafness occurs from catarrh. Inflammation at the base of the left lung. Sulphur will often help to clear up a residual consolidation or congestion in the lung after the acute symptoms have cleared up but there is failure of resolution.

## Gastrointestinal

Desire for sweet, *fat,* butter, *stimulants.*

Empty, sinking feeling about an hour before lunch (11 a.m.).

Feels hungry, but on sitting down have a poor appetite, but marked *thirst.*

Flatulent distension with burning and colic.

Early morning *diarrhoea* which drives him out of bed, with burning stool, redness and excoriation round anus, and congested haemorrhoids.

Bad taste on waking, ulceration of the mouth, chronic sore throat which has a purplish appearance.

## Genito-urinary

Urging and burning on urination, eruptions on genitals, burning leucorrhoea. In uterine haemorrhage or abortion Sulphur is often needed to follow; Aconite, Belladonna or Sabina as acute remedies.

Dysmenorrhoea in a Sulphur patient. *Hot flushes* at menopause (Lachesis, Sepia).

## Rheumatic

Rheumatic conditions if general symptoms fit, especially if hands and feet burn.

Low back pain on rising, turning in bed.

Tendency to bedsores or corns and bunions on slight pressure.

## Sleep

Restless and disturbed, wakes at 3 a.m. and cannot sleep again, dreams, hot in bed, throws off bedclothes.

General aggravation *at night.*

## Other useful indications

Complementary to Aconite – its acute remedy.

Sulphur, Calcarea Carb. and Lycopodium follow each other well, in that order.

Measles with a marked purplish rash.

When symptoms occur as a result of suppression of eruptions.

When well-indicated remedies fail to act.

Where there are few symptoms to prescribe on.

## SYPHILINUM (Lueticum)

A nosode prepared from a chancre.

Mention has been made in the text about Hahnemann's Miasms, syphilis being one. Patients may develop a wide variety of symptoms, either from a previous infection or due to hereditary traits passed down from ancestors who have had syphilis. It is not a remedy to use in the active phase. As well as having a variety of symptoms and signs there are a number of physical characteristics associated with this remedy.

Thin, dwarf-like persons, with prominent forehead, retroussé nose, ears which tend to be small, or to stick out or be out of alignment, baldness, shining dry emaciated skin, drooping eyelids and shotty glands.

Of value where there are enlarged lymph glands, ulcers, contractures, abscesses, ovarian tumours.

Accident prone, tendency to epilepsy, haemorrhage, hemiplegia.

Great weakness and exhaustion in the mornings.

AGGRAVATION of symptoms at NIGHT, at the SEA, in WINTER; better from motion, and in mountainous country.

GRADUAL onset and disappearance of symptoms.

### Mentals
Suicidal, depressed.
Constant inclination to *wash his hands*.
Sleeplessness in the elderly.

### Eyes
Ulcers of the cornea, keratitis.

### Gastrointestinal
Craving for alcohol, and cold food.
Salivation, cracked fissured tongue.
Prolapse of rectum and piles.

### Genital
Acrid leucorrhoea, scanty menses.
Depression at the menopause.

### Other symptoms
Pains tend to run in a line – up or down. Patients are *not* sensitive to pain.
If ill tends to lie covered up.

## THUJA

This is Burnett's great remedy for the effects of vaccination, either where there has been a bad reaction or failure to react, or where the patient is never well since.

Hahnemann's great remedy in Sycosis or following gonorrhoea. These patients look sickly, pale, waxy; are easily exhausted.

CHILLY, sensitive to DAMP, have CHRONIC CATARRH or WARTY GROWTHS. On exposure of the body to warm air there is shivering all over, warm air feels cold.

Profuse SWEAT on UNCOVERED parts; sweetish smelling sweat.

### Mentals
Anxious, indisposed to do anything, weeps easily, especially at music. Irritable, may act or talk hurriedly.

Mistakes in reading or writing. Speaks slowly as if at a loss for words. Prolonged thoughtfulness at the merest trifles.

*Fixed ideas:* as if the body were brittle and would break; as if the legs were made of wood; as if a live animal were in the abdomen.

### Headache
Accompanied by vertigo, neuralgias – sensation as if a nail were driven into the temple, or a tight band was round the head.

Headaches worse on waking or at bedtime.

Worse in heat, better in the open air.

### Eyes
Conjunctivitis – especially gonorrhoeal.

### Respiratory
Post-nasal catarrh and pharyngitis, affections of the mucous membranes, foul smelling discharges, polyps.

Asthma worse in damp. May follow Arsenicum after the acute attack.

### Gastrointestinal
Carious roots of teeth, pyorrhoea, gums swollen and inflamed.

Tongue red and painful; sweetish taste in the mouth.

A remedy to antidote excessive tea drinking.

Eructations, nausea and wind.

Anal fissures, piles and warty growths, painful.

### Genito-urinary
Pain anywhere causes frequency of micturition – pale, watery urine.

Sweat of the genitalia, offensive.

Gonorrhoea, warty like excrescences, soft, sensitive and burning.

Periods early with severe left ovarian pain.
In the male, urethritis, prostatitis.

**Skin**
Scaly eruptions, pustular eruptions, herpes zoster, warts.
Effects of smallpox or vaccination.

**Sleep**
Wakes early and cannot sleep afterwards.
Dreams of falling from a height.

**Other symptoms**
Rheumatism and arthritis, especially when related to gonorrhoea or to leucorrhoea or pelvic symptoms.
Always worse in damp weather; foul smelling sweats.

Thuja is often the chronic remedy related to Arsenicum, especially in asthma.
Related to other Sycotic remedies Natrum Sulph., Nitric Acid, Medorrhinum.

## TUBERCULINUM BOVINUM (Prepared from tuberculous abscess or sputum)

This remedy should always be considered where there is a family history of TB, or a past history in the patient of tuberculous infection.

It is a remedy of intermittent fever – cases that relapse or where a well-selected remedy acts and yet does not hold.

Recurring colds and coughs on the least exposure. Sharp pains in the left upper lung.

Loves wind and open air. Upset in a close atmosphere; sensitive to damp.

Periodicity 7, 21, 28 days – periodic chronic headache.

DESIRE FOR CHANGE, house, travel, decoration, never satisfied in one place, cosmopolitan. Children may run away from home. Symptoms change: sudden onset, sudden cessation.

### Mentals
Hopeless, aversion to mental work, anxiety in the evening, fear of dogs. Temper *tantrums* in children.

### Gastrointestinal
*Desires:* salt, cold milk, alcohol – thirsty.
*Averse:* meat.
Emaciation while eating well – eats in the night, but also loss of appetite.
Constipation or chronic diarrhoea in the morning (Sulphur).

### Genital
Menses early, profuse and long; also amenorrhoea, dysmenorrhoea.

### Limbs
Wandering pains in limbs and joints, stiff on first moving, better from continued motion (Rhus Tox.). Worse on standing.

### Sleep
Dreams, waking 5 a.m., clammy sweats especially in night.

## BACILLINUM (Heath's and Burnett's preparation from TB lung, containing bacilli)

Deep-seated severe headache.
Cough with easy expectoration; sharp pain in the left scapula.
Pains in the glands of the neck.
Aching in teeth – sensitive to cold air.
Inflammatory conditions of the eyelids.
Restless, disturbed sleep.
Windy dyspepsia.

## VERATRUM ALBUM (White Hellebore)

This was one of Hahnemann's cholera remedies, along with Camphor and Cuprum.

Veratrum is characterised by COLLAPSE with prostration, COLD-NESS, blueness, and PROFUSE DISCHARGES. It also has marked mental symptoms.

### Mentals
A violent remedy in states of mental illness.

Delirium, destructive – wants to tear or destroy, tears at his clothes or pulls them off (like Hyoscyamus).

Religious frenzy, exhorts people to repent.

Screams with obscene songs, and lascivious or amorous behaviour. Fear of death or being damned.

### Coldness
This is marked with shivering or rigors, *cold sweat* on the forehead. Skin cold and blue, and yet there is *aggravation from heat.*

### Copious discharges
This may be vomit, diarrhoea, sweat, urine, or salivation.

This loss of fluid causes collapse, fainting, rapid exhaustion and prostration, the skin becomes cold and blue, the face looks drawn and ill. Cramps may then develop (a typical Cholera picture).

### Fainting
May occur with less severe causes, from emotional stress or exertion.

The pulse is slow and weak and the blood pressure low.

It may be of value in cardiac cases.

Constipation may occur with large, hard stools, with colic, urging and again cold sweat and faintness.

### Pain
Neuralgias of all kinds, headaches and *dysmenorrhoea,* where there is prostration, cold sweats and vomiting. *Heat* always *aggravates* and the patient is restless.

## ZINCUM

An antipsoric remedy indicated in feeble constitutions.

Nervous, excitable, sensitive to noises or talking, with tremblings, twitchings and jerking of muscles.

Incessant violent FIDGETING OF THE FEET or lower limbs.

Yet there is lack of vitality, 'brain fag', slowness of mind – must repeat the question before answering.

Anaemia.

### Generals
*Chilly* – sensitive to cold.

Symptoms from failure of something to come out. Examples are: where a discharge or eruption has not appeared, a child is restless, cries in sleep and rolls his head from side to side – once a rash emerges he is much improved; where the patient cannot expectorate but feels better when he does; where menstruation is of late onset, and the flow relieves (as in Lachesis).

### Gastrointestinal
Hunger about 11–12 a.m. (Sulphur) – greedy.

Aggravation from wine or stimulants.

Sluggish bowel and bladder.

### Rheumatic
Aching weariness in the nape of the neck, dorsal and lumbar spine worse on sitting, first rising, better from moving. (Rhus Tox. is often in the sacral region.)

Burning feeling along the spine.

# HOMOEOPATHIC BOOKS FOR STUDY

*Introduction to the Principles and Practice of Homoeopathy*   C. E. Wheeler and J. D. Kenyon

*Homoeopathic Drug Pictures*   M. L. Tyler

*Leaders in Homoeopathic Therapeutics*   E. B. Nash

*Keynotes of Leading Remedies*   M. C. Allen

*The Prescriber*   J. H. Clarke

*The Patient not the Cure*   M. Blackie

*Homoeopathy*   C. Ruthven Mitchell (An excellent historical book.)

*Lectures on Homoeopathic Philosophy*   J. T. Kent

*Materia Medica with Repertory*   W. Boericke (Useful reference book.)

*Principles and Art of Cure by Homoeopathy*   H. A. Roberts

*How to use the Repertory*   G. I. Bidwell

*The Organon of the Rational System of Medicine*   Samuel Hahnemann

*The Healing Art of Homoeopathy*   E. C. Hamlyn (A modern interpretation of the *Organon*.)

*Homoeopathic Prescribing*   N. J. Pratt

*Homoeopathy in Practice*   D. M. Borland, edited by K. M. Priestman (1981)

*Lectures on Homoeopathic Materia Medica*   J. T. Kent

*Repertory of Homoeopathic Materia Medica*   J. T. Kent

*Dictionary of Practical Materia Medica*   J. H. Clarke, 3 volumes

# BOOKLETS AND SMALL BOOKS USEFUL FOR BEGINNERS OR LAYMEN

*Elements of Homoeopathy*    D. M. Gibson

*First Aid Homoeopathy*    D. M. Gibson

*Homoeopathy – an Introductory Guide*    A. C. G. Ross

*Homoeopathy, Born 1810*    R. Livingstone

*Essentials of Homoeopathic Prescribing*    H. Fergie Woods

*Children's Types*    D. M. Borland

*Influenza*    D. M. Borland

*Pneumonias*    D. M. Borland

*Digestive Drugs*    D. M. Borland

*Homoeopathy for Mother and Infant*    D. M. Borland

*Pointers to the Common Remedies, 1–9*    M. L. Tyler

Especially useful are:
1 – Colds, acute chest
2 – Stomach, digestive
5 – Infectious fevers


*Introducing Homoeopathy into General Practice*    R. A. F. Jack

*Comparative Value of Symptoms in the Selection of the Remedy*    R. Gibson Miller

*Relationship of Remedies*    R. Gibson Miller

*Study of Kent's Repertory*    M. Tyler

*The Bowel Nosodes*    John Paterson

# GLOSSARY OF SPECIALISED TERMS IN HOMOEOPATHY

AGGRAVATION A temporary worsening of symptoms sometimes following the taking of a remedy, usually succeeded by a distinct improvement in the patient's condition.

CONSTITUTIONAL REMEDY A remedy prescribed on the basis of the temperament, character and general reactions of the patient (their constitutional type) as well as the local symptoms of disease.

DRUG PICTURE A summary of the symptoms, mental states and pathological changes that a substance is capable of causing (and treating) in human beings.

HOMOEOPATHY The system of medicine developed by Samuel Hahnemann invoking the principle that effective and non-toxic treatment may be given by using substances that can cause symptoms in the healthy similar to those the patient is suffering. This is summarised as 'similia similibus curentur' or 'let likes be treated by likes'. (Homoios — like, pathos — suffering: Greek.)

MATERIA MEDICA The homoeopathic pharmacopoeia; a list of remedies with their associated symptoms and uses.

MIASMS Conditions which may be acquired or inherited, and which have been postulated as the basic underlying cause of chronic and recurrent disease conditions. For example, Hahnemann considered all chronic disease to be manifestations of three miasms, syphilis, sycosis and psora, acting singly or in combination, and amenable to treatment by the appropriate remedies.

MODALITIES Those factors that qualify a particular symptom, e.g. pain worse from motion, better from local heat. Aggravating factors are often abbreviated to $<$ and ameliorating factors to $>$. In above example: pain $<$ motion, $>$ heat.

NOSODES Remedies derived from the products of disease (sputum, pus, etc.), diseased tissue or pathogenic organisms. The bowel nosodes are derived from culture of intestinal bacteria.

POLYCRESTS Certain remedies which are very well-known and which have a wide range of clinical application, often being prescribed on the patient's constitutional type.

POTENCY Most homoeopathic remedies are used in potency; in other words, the substances have been put through the process of serial dilution with succussion (or trituration if insoluble) at each stage of dilution. This is potentisation and may be carried out with dilutions of one-in-ten – decimal scale, or one-in-a-hundred – the centesimal scale. A potency involving six dilutions on the decimal scale is written 6x (6DH in Continental Europe), while six dilutions on the centesimal scale is 6c or just 6 (6CH in Continental Europe).

Low potency 1x up to 12x (6c).

High potency 30c, 200c, 1M (1000c), 10M.

PROVING The testing of a substance on healthy volunteers (provers) who take repeated doses and record in detail any symptoms produced. (Prüfen – to test: German, from Latin probare.)

REPERTORY An index of drug symptoms, each heading or rubric listing those drugs known to cause the symptom. Often the remedies are printed in different type to denote the prominence of the symptom in provings and clinical experience; from black type, where the symptom comes through strongly, through italics to ordinary type. Hence 'black letter symptoms'.

SIMILIMUM The single remedy that best fits the total symptom picture.

SPOT AND SPECIFIC PRESCRIBING This is a prescribing method, which, although based on the principle of similars, pays more attention to the local, particular signs of a disease, and less to the general response shown by the individual, e.g. Arnica which is almost specific for bruising. Certain remedies also have organ specificities, and are prescribed on a pathological basis.

SUCCUSSION Violent shaking at each stage of dilution in the preparation of a potency. Traditionally the container is hit rhythmically against leather or the heel of the hand, but succussion is now usually mechanical.

TINCTURE Remedies in liquid form, normally with a mixture of alcohol and water as solvent. The remedy in its most concentrated form is known as the mother tincture, designated $\phi$, and it is from this that the potencies are made by serial dilution and succussion.

TRITURATION Prolonged grinding with an inert base, usually lactose, in the preparation of a potency from an insoluble substance.

VITAL FORCE OR DYNAMIS This term was used by Hahnemann to describe the innate recuperative power within the human body, which he envisaged could be stimulated by the homoeopathic potency. In disease this vital force is disordered and the remedy helps to correct this.

# Questions for Reflection and Discussion

## PRINCIPLES AND PHILOSOPHY

What are the basic principles of homoeopathic prescribing?

What are the sources of homoeopathic remedies, and how are they prepared?

What is a potency? Can you indicate the commonly used potencies and when they are used?

List the main headings to be followed in taking a homoeopathic history in a chronic case.

What is the homoeopathic doctor's concept of chronic disease, its origins and progression, and what do we mean by 'directions of cure'?

What is meant by 'proving'? What other sources of information are used in compiling a homoeopathic materia medica?

It is often said that the second prescription is more difficult than the first. What would you ask at the second interview, and what possible alternatives are there for the next prescription?

What is meant by the prescribing of similars? Can you think of any instances of this principle in conventional medicine?

In what forms are homoeopathic remedies dispensed? How do you choose, and how would you give the remedy to the patient – in what dose, how often?

Describe your ideas of possible fields of research in homoeopathy, bearing in mind the difficulty of individual prescribing in the double blind situation.

Write short notes on the following: a) General symptom. b) Particular symptom. c) Polycrest. d) Aggravation. e) Time modality.

What is meant by 'pathological' and 'organ' prescribing? Give five examples.

What is the importance of Past History and Family History in prescribing a homoeopathic remedy? Give illustrations.

A patient's personal reaction to environment and events (e.g. grief, fright, resentment) can often be altered by homoeopathic remedies. Name five remedies used in these circumstances, and what you would hope to achieve.

The appearance and behaviour of a patient is often helpful in selecting a remedy. Illustrate this with five common remedies.

## MATERIA MEDICA

Describe the common accident and injury remedies and indications for their use.

Silica and Calcarea Carb. are both chilly remedies – compare and contrast their symptom pictures.

Give the indications for selecting three of the influenza remedies.

A child presents with a fever. What symptoms and signs would you look for in selecting a remedy in acute disease? Describe three acute remedies.

What features differentiate Sepia and Natrum Mur.?

How would you tackle a case of asthma from a homoeopathic point of view, both in the acute phase and in the longer term, illustrating with some remedy pictures?

Give details of six remedies of value in acute sore throats or laryngitis.

Compare and contrast Pulsatilla and Phosphorus.

A patient presents with symptoms of peptic ulcer. Describe how you would take the case history, with distinguishing modalities, illustrating your answer with remedies.

Describe a typical Lycopodium patient and his symptom complex.

In what ways does the picture of Nux Vomica differ from that of Lycopodium?

A patient presents with diarrhoea and colic. Describe some suitable remedies for this, with modalities.

Describe the symptom picture you associate with Phosphoric Acid.

Describe your approach to a child with eczema, and give details of the possible remedies you might prescribe.

Describe the symptom picture you associate with Sulphur and Graphites. Compare the similarities and differences.

What remedies would you think to prescribe in acute cystitis? Give details of the symptom pictures in these remedies.

Sepia and Lilium Tigrinum have some common similarities. What are these, and how do they also differ?

What do you know of the value of Causticum in respiratory and urinary complaints?

Three remedies often used in patients with leucorrhoea are Nitric Acid, Kreosotum and Hydrastis. Can you distinguish the leading indications?

Describe the modalities that would help you distinguish between four of the remedies for angina.

Describe the pictures suggesting Carbo Veg., Kali Carb., and Apis in cardiac failure.

What is the picture of Lachesis?

Describe and compare four remedies used in acute headache.

How would you approach a migraine case from a homoeopathic point of view?

Describe two remedies of value in the preventive treatment of migraine or chronic headaches.

Recurring sinusitis is a frequent problem in practice. What remedies might be used in the acute phase and also to reduce the catarrhal state? Give the symptoms in four remedies which would help you to prescribe in such a case.

Compare and contrast Rhus Tox., Bryonia and Causticum in the treatment of rheumatic disease.

Modalities are often very valuable in treating rheumatism or arthritis. List a few with their indicated remedies.

What symptoms do you associate with Ferrum Met. and Rhododendron in rheumatism?

Nash describes four restless and violent remedies. Can you list these and describe their chief features?

Aurum Met. and Natrum Sulph. are both remedies for depression. Describe their leading symptoms and indications.

Elderly patients can be helped by homoeopathic remedies. What symptoms would suggest the use of Anacardium, Conium and Baryta Carb.?

Give a concise description of the types of children and their main presenting symptoms which would make you prescribe Calc. Carb., Silica and Phosphorus.

A child is brought with a history of recurring coughs, colds and wheezes. What questions would you ask the mother and what three remedies might help? Give their symptom pictures.

Compare the differences between two remedies used in children, characterised by burning – Sulphur and Arsenicum Alb.

What are the indications for the use of the bowel nosodes Morgan Co. and Sycotic Co.?

Describe the leading features of the two nosodes Medorrhinum and Syphilinum.

# Remedy Index

Page numbers in bold type refer to a full drug picture in Section III of this book.

# Subject Index

# THE TRUE HEALING ART

# List of Pharmacies and Companies in the United States and Canada that Can Supply Homeopathic Remedies

(Courtesy of the National Center for Homeopathy, Falls Church, Virginia 22042)

## CALIFORNIA

City Pharmacy
1435 State Street
Santa Barbara, CA 93101

College Pharmacy
90 N. Ashwood Avenue
Ventura, CA 93003

Horton and Converse
621 West Pico Boulevard
Los Angeles, CA 90015

Mylans Homeopathic Pharmacy
222 O'Farrell Street
San Francisco, CA 94102

Nutri-Dyn
717 S. Bristol Ave.
Los Angeles, CA 90049

Santa Monica Drug
1513 Fourth Street
Santa Monica, CA 90401

Standard Homeopathic
Company
436 West 8th Avenue
Los Angeles, CA 90014

Village Drug Store
Ojai, CA 93023

## ILLINOIS

Ehrhart and Karl
17 N. Wabash Ave.
Chicago, IL 60602

## MARYLAND

Washington Homeopathic
Pharmacy
4914 Delray Avenue
Bethesda, MD 20014

## MISSOURI

Luyties Pharmacal Company
4200 Laclede Avenue
St. Louis, MO 63108

## NEW JERSEY

Humphreys Pharmacal Company
63 Meadow Road
Rutherford, NJ 07070

## NEW YORK

Keihl Pharmacy, Inc.
109 Third Avenue
New York, NY 10003

Weleda, Inc.
841 South Main Street
Spring Valley, NY 10977

## PENNSYLVANIA

Boericke and Tafel, Inc.
1011 Arch Street
Philadelphia, PA 19107

John A. Borneman and Sons
1208 Amosland Road
Norwood, PA 19074

## VIRGINIA

Annandale Apothecary
7023 Little River Turnpike
Annandale, VA 22003

## CANADA

D. L. Thompson Homeopathic
  Supplies
844 Yonge Street
Toronto 5, Ontario
Canada M4W 2H1